To contact the publisher, visit: www.representpublishing.com
To contact the author, visit: www.littleapplelove.com

ISBN 979-8-9922605-6-4
Printed in the United States of America

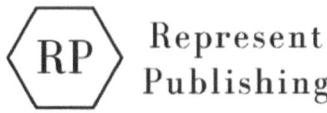

Edited and Formatted by Represent Publishing
Cover Design by BEDESIGNS.CA
Photography by Cailee Nicole Photography and Holly C Walsh

DISCLAIMER NOTICE

The recipes, tips, and information presented in this book are for educational and informational purposes only and are not intended to diagnose, treat, cure, or prevent any disease. The content is based on the personal experiences and research of Little Apple Love, LLC and Holly C Walsh, and should not be considered medical advice.

We are not licensed medical professionals, and any information provided should not be used as a substitute for consultation with qualified healthcare providers. Always seek the advice of your physician or other licensed health professional before making changes to your diet, lifestyle, or wellness practices.

By using this book, you acknowledge and agree that you are solely responsible for your own health decisions and for any outcomes resulting from your use of the information provided.

**Little Apple Love, LLC and Holly C Walsh disclaim all liability for any adverse effects or consequences resulting from the use or application of any content in this publication.

THE
JUICY
TRUTH

THE JUICY TRUTH

HOLLY C WALSH

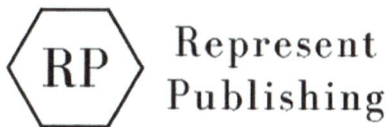

Represent Publishing

To the souls I encountered at the café . . . some of you were pure juice, others more like the pulp I had to strain out. Grateful for all of it.

TABLE OF CONTENTS

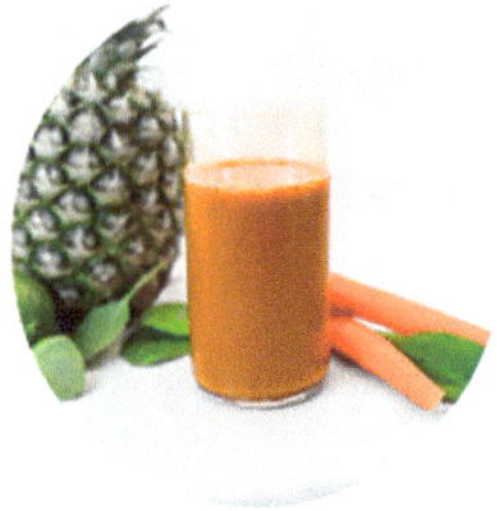

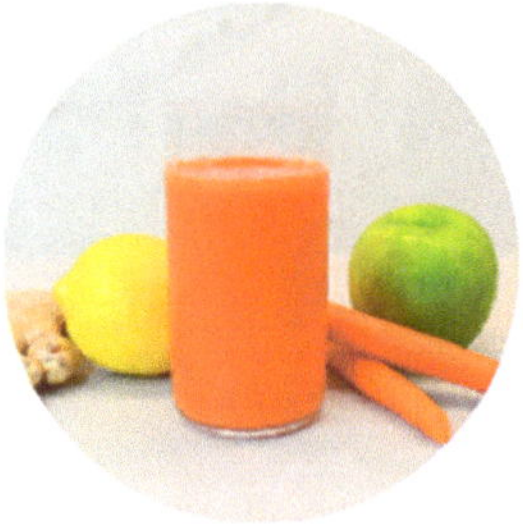

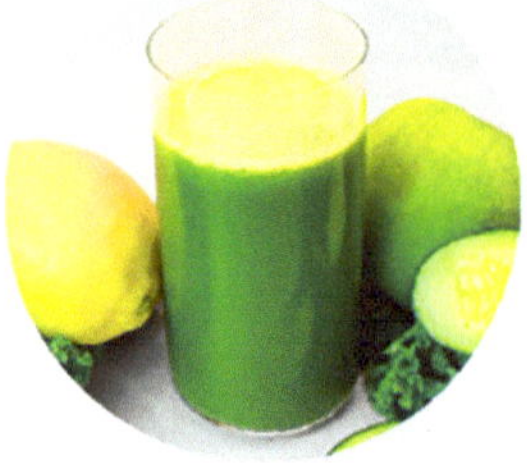

fresh pressed juice

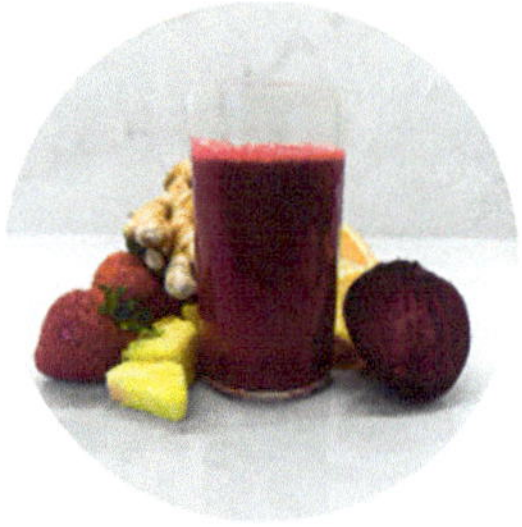

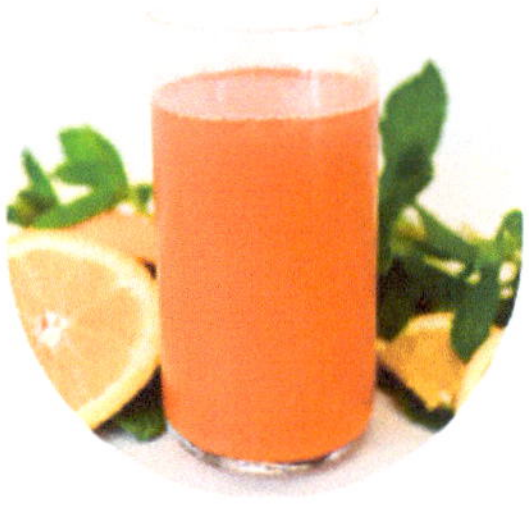

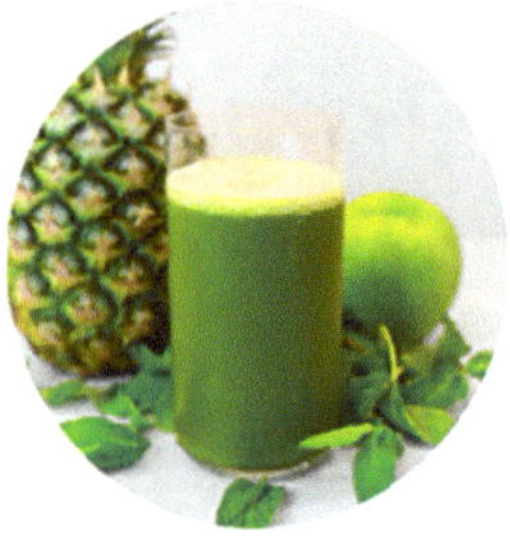

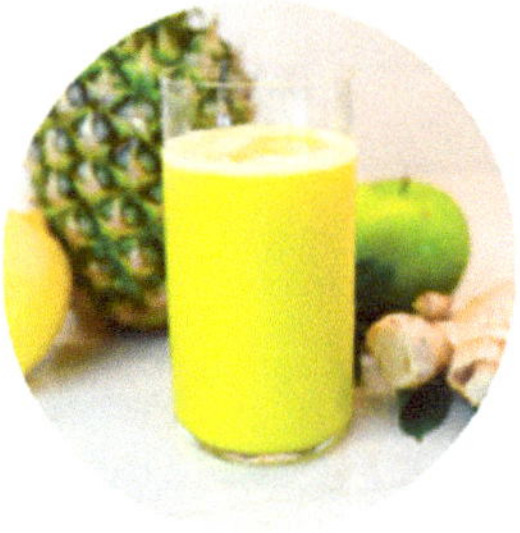

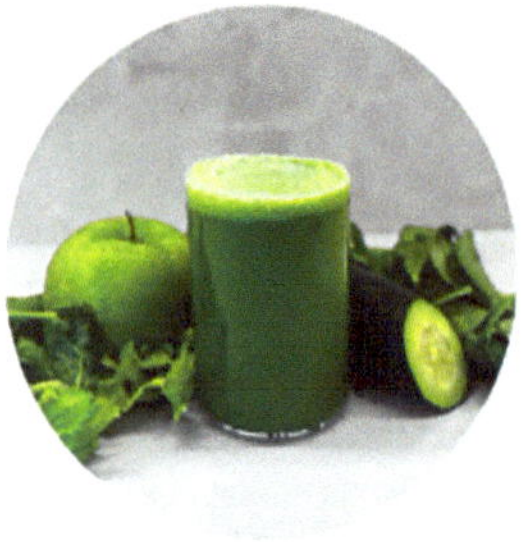

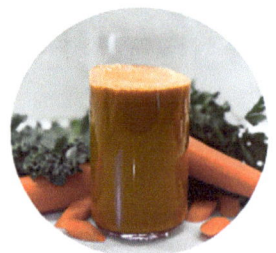
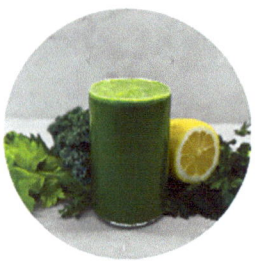
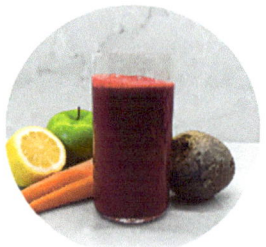
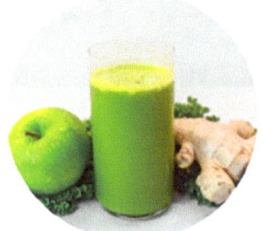

corecleanse

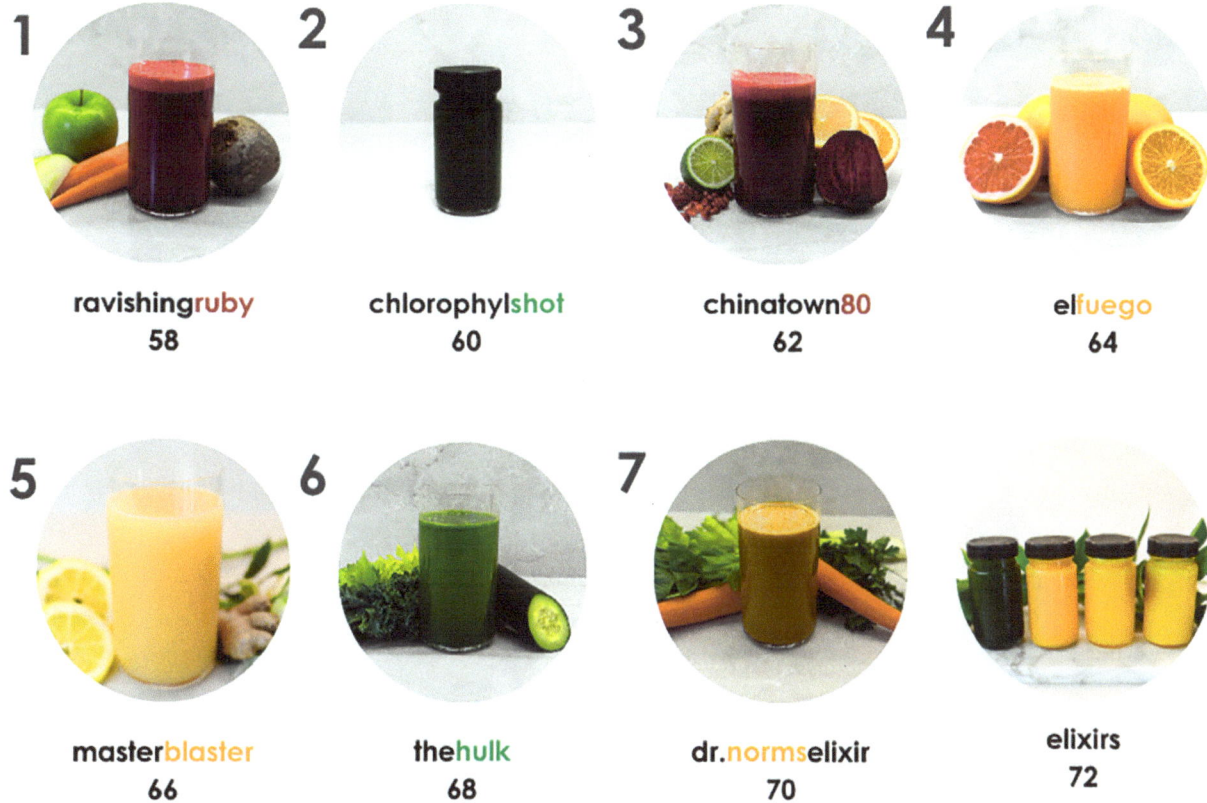

1
ravishingruby
58

2
chlorophylshot
60

3
chinatown80
62

4
elfuego
64

5
masterblaster
66

6
thehulk
68

7
dr.normselixir
70

elixirs
72

TABLE OF CONTENTS

smoothies

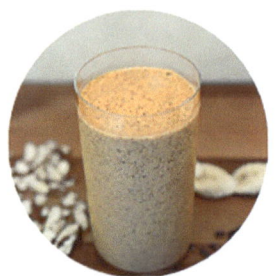
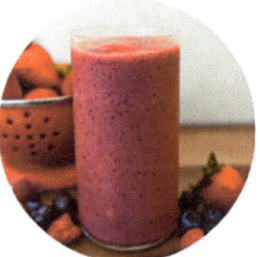
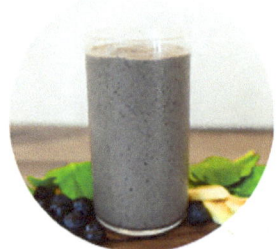
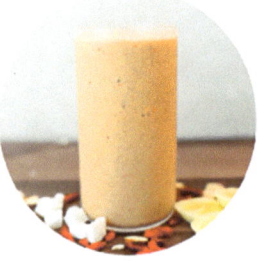
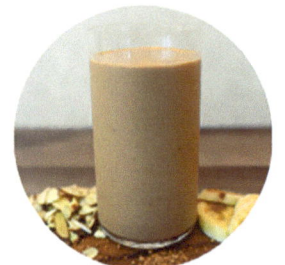
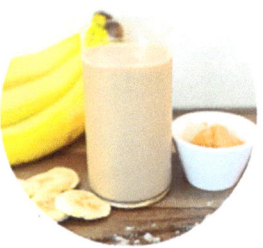
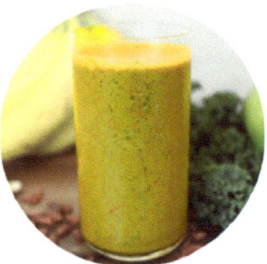
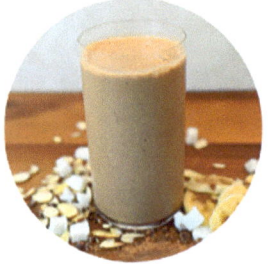
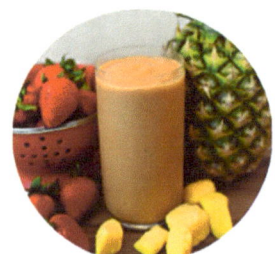
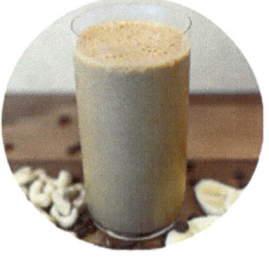
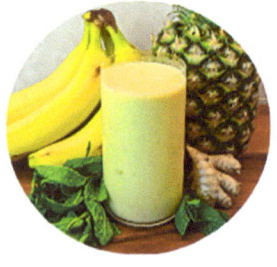
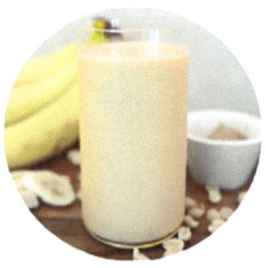

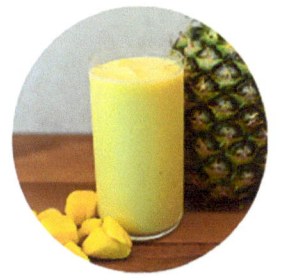

pinappleparadise
104

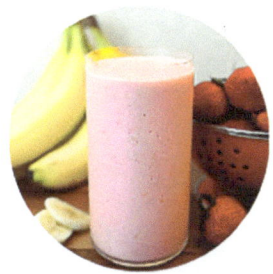

scrumptiousstrawberry
106

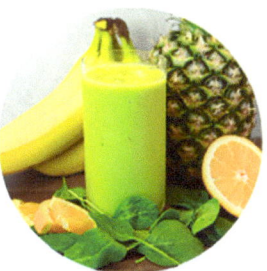

thedutchess
108

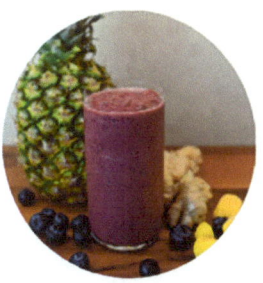

tropicalblast
110

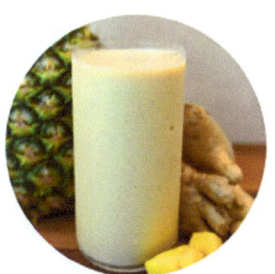

tropicalsunrise
112

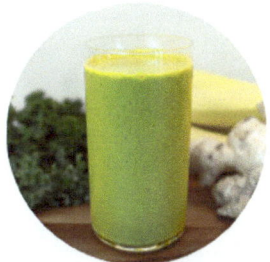

you'vegotkale
114

TABLE OF CONTENTS

açaí & smoothie bowls

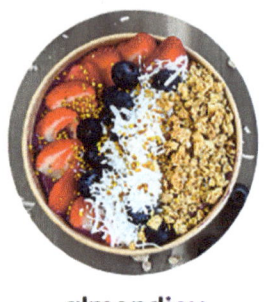
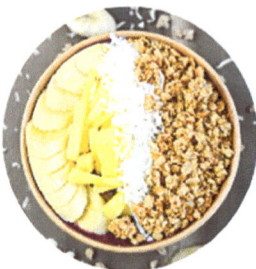
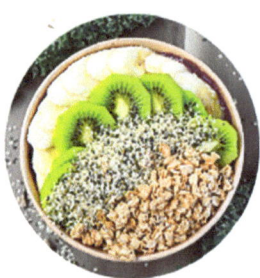
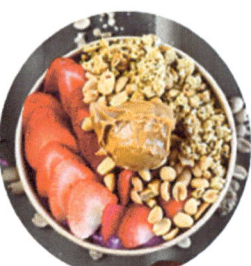
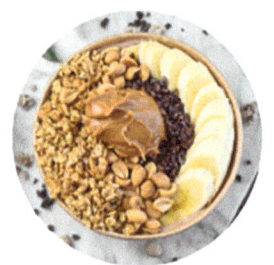
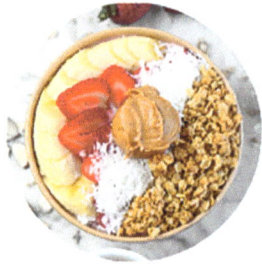
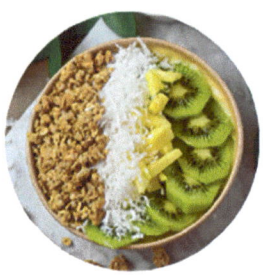
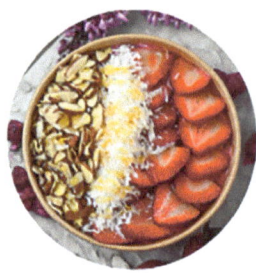

mocktails

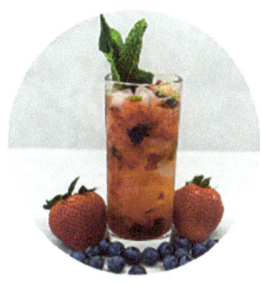

berryfojito
142

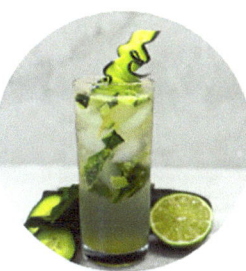

cucumberbreeze
144

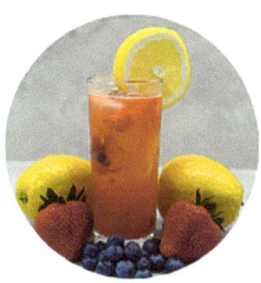

lemonberrysparkler
146

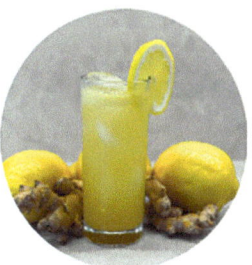

lemongingerfizz
148

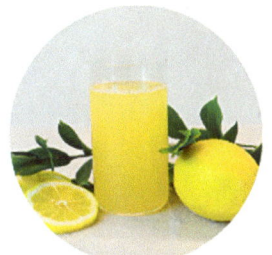

lemonlulu
150

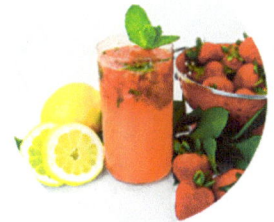

strawberrymintlemonade
152

TABLE OF CONTENTS

bites & delights

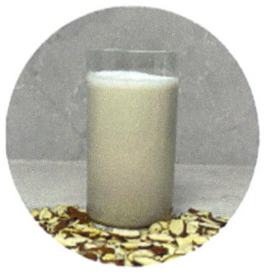
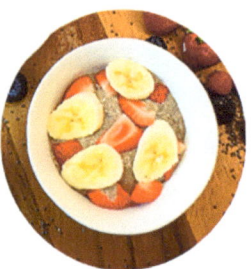
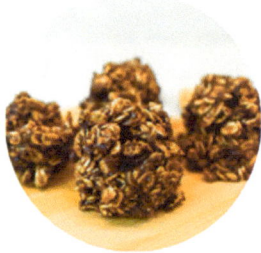
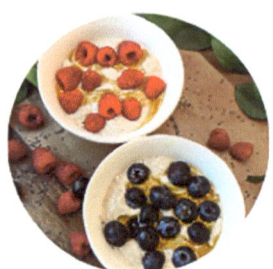
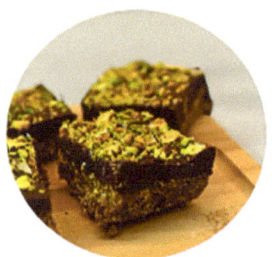
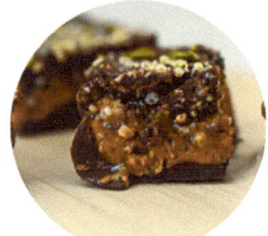
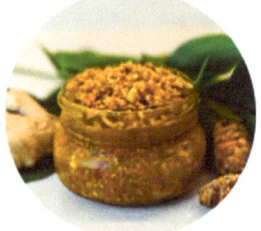
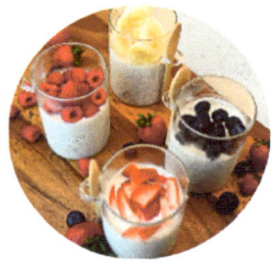
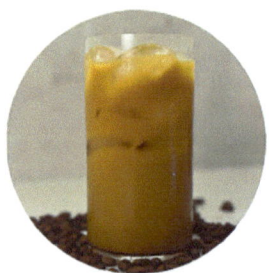
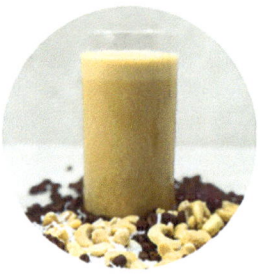

INTRODUCTION

Well, here we are. I finally did it! I wrote my book. My goal is, and always has been, to help people lead healthier lives. My motto: Healthy doesn't have to be hard.

Most of the recipes compiled in this book are customer favorites from when I owned Little Apple™ Café in Woodstock, NY.

How did Little Apple™ Café come to be?

It was originally called Little Apple™, which was a long-time staple in Woodstock, NY. My son and I would frequent the spot whenever we were in town. One evening, my husband and I were sitting on the couch and he was reading through Craigslist ads. One caught his eye, and he said, "Here you go, juice bar for sale in Woodstock. That's all you."

With my experience in the fitness industry, education in becoming a health coach, and dedication to helping people transform their lives, I knew this was an opportunity I had to jump on. So, we made the call, and the rest is history. After an internal clean-up and a menu revival, we were officially off and running in October 2019.

When COVID hit in March 2020, we were the first restaurant in the area to close the doors and transition to takeout only. Luckily, we had a wonderful outside patio with a window that we made our "TO GO" order and pickup window. As time when on, and we got busier and busier, we expanded to utilize the entire inside for production.

After 5 years, we closed the doors on the café, but the recipes, customers, and experiences have left a lasting impact. We're so thankful and appreciative of all the time we spent there.

The Juicy Truth is my thank you to the loyal customers who loved all our products. This book is a way to keep Little Apple™ alive without being tied to a location. These recipes have been made thousands of times and are near and dear to my heart. I now give you my creations, and I hope it inspires you to choose healthy options.

If you were a long-time customer, I hope you find joy in continuing the Little Apple™ Café recipes in the comfort of your own home. If you're just discovering Little Apple™, welcome. We hope you enjoy these creations.

Peace, Love, and Juice,
Holly

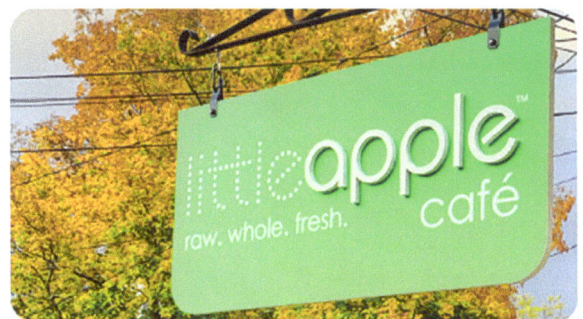
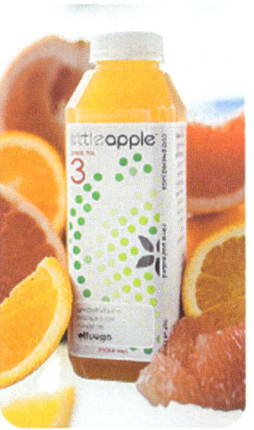
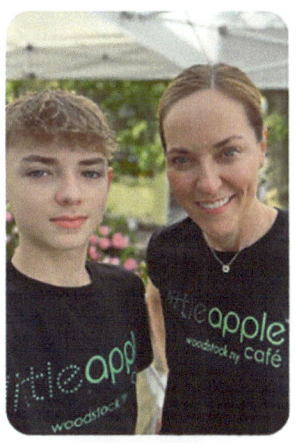
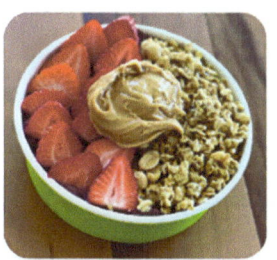
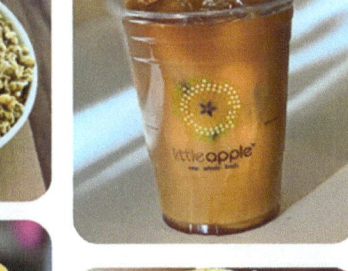
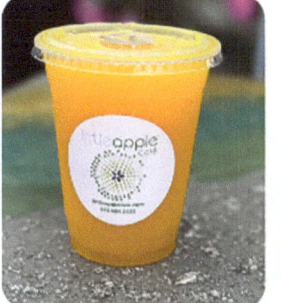
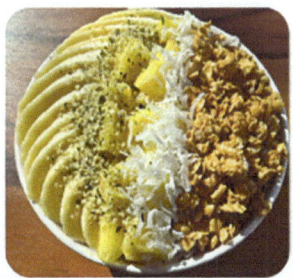
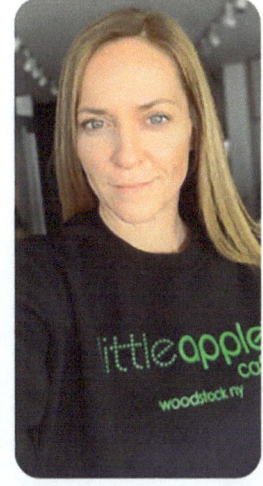
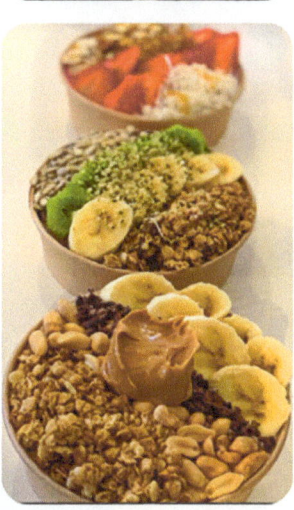
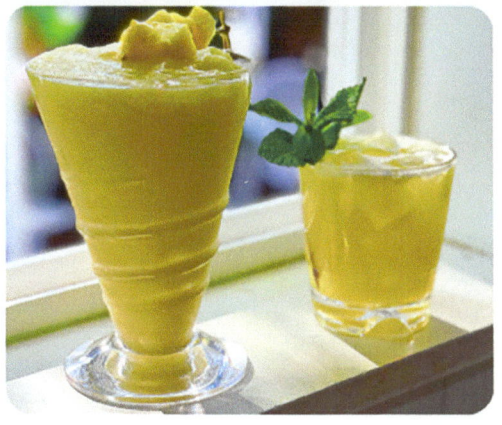
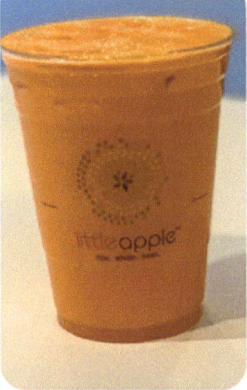
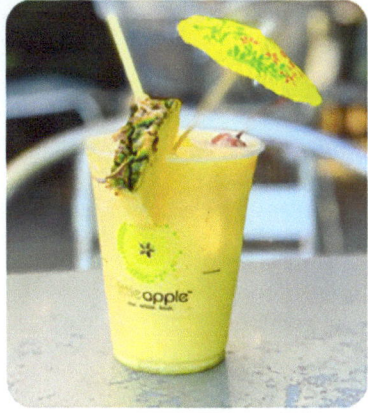

CONVERSIONS

1 tablespoon = 3 teaspoons

8 tablespoons = 1/2 cup or 4 fluid ounce

8 fluid ounce = 1 cup

1 pint = 2 cups

1 quart = 32 fluid ounce

4 quarts = 1 gallon

1 gallon = 128 fluid ounce

1 fluid ounce = 30 milliliter

1 pound = 16 weighted ounce

KITCHEN TOOLS

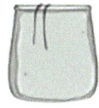 Cheesecloth/ Nutmilk bag strainer

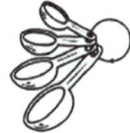 Measuring spoons

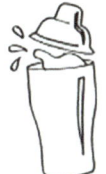 Cocktail shaker

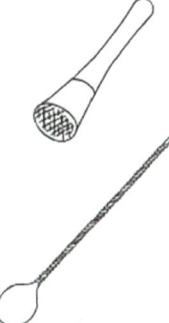 Muddler

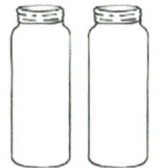 Glass bottles for juices

Long-handled bar spoon

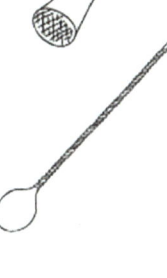 High quality blender

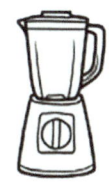 Silicone spatula set

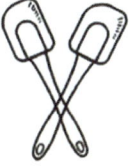 High quality juicer

Silicone storage bag or container for frozen fruit

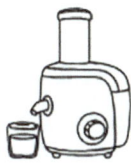 Jigger

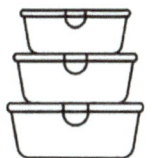 Strainer for rinsing fruits and vegetables

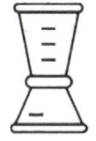

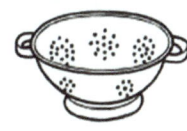

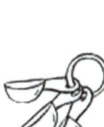 Measuring cups

SHOPPING LIST

Fresh Fruits & Veggies

- Carrots
- Celery
- Cilantro
- Cucumber
- Ginger
- Granny Smith Apple
- Grapefruit
- Kale
- Lemon
- Lime
- Mint
- Orange
- Parsley
- Pineapple
- Red Beets
- Spinach
- Turmeric

Fresh Fruit for Bowl Toppings

- Banana
- Blueberries
- Kiwi
- Pineapple
- Strawberries

Frozen Fruits

- Apple
- Açaí
- Banana
- Blueberries
- Coconut Meat
- Mango
- Pineapple
- Pitaya (Dragonfruit)
- Raspberries
- Strawberries

Smoothie & Bowl Liquid

- Coconut Water
- Iced Coffee
- Unsweetened Almond Milk
- Unsweetened Coconut Milk
- Unsweetened Oat Milk

Pantry Staples for Recipes

- Agave
- Almonds (whole & raw)
- Almonds (sliced & raw)
- Almond Butter (unsweetened)
- Bee Pollen
- Cacao Powder
- Cacao Nibs
- Cayenne extract
- Cinnamon
- Chia Seeds
- Chlorophyl
- Coconut cubes
- Coconut Flakes
- Dates (pitted or seedless)
- Flax Oil
- Goji Berries
- Granola
- Hemp Protein
- Hemp Seeds
- Honey
- Maca Powder
- Maple Syrup
- Moringa Powder
- Peanuts (raw)
- Peanut Butter (unsweetened)
- Spirulina
- Vanilla
- Vegan Chocolate Protein
- Vegan Vanilla Protein

TIPS

- Holly loves Ceylon cinnamon. It has a milder, more delicate flavor.
- Buy dry or fresh coconut cubes. Health food stores usually have fresh, or you can get dried online.
- Holly's favorite protein powder is Truvani Plant Based Protein Powder

PREPARING PRODUCE

The best way to wash produce is to give it a good rinse with cool running water, even if it has a peel or outer skin. For things like apples, carrots, and cucumbers, you can scrub them gently with a vegetable brush to remove dirt. For leafy greens, like spinach or lettuce, it's helpful to soak them in a bowl of water and then rinse them thoroughly under running water to get rid of any dirt or residue.

Some people also use a vinegar solution (1 part vinegar to 3 parts water) to help remove bacteria but it's not necessary unless you're concerned about specific contamination. Just be sure to rinse again with plain water afterward.

You can also use a veggie wash of your choice. You can put the fruits or veggies in a bowl or sink. Spray the veggies and let sit for a few minutes and then rinse. Holly finds veggie wash to work well on berries.

Apples
Remove the sticker, wash and rinse. Cut into quarters and remove the seeds.

Banana
Peel the skin, break into 1-inch pieces, put in a freezer bag, and lay flat.

Beets & Carrots
Cut off the ends slightly, then wash and rinse thoroughly.

Celery
Pull the bunches apart, wash, and rinse thoroughly, ensuring all dirt is removed.

Citrus
Peel the skin with a knife or peel before use.

Cucumbers
Wash and rinse thoroughly

Ginger, Turmeric, Parsley, Mint, Cilantro
Rinse under cold water before use.

Kale/Spinach
Soak in the sink with a wash solution for 10 minutes, then rinse thoroughly.

Pineapple
Peel the skin completely.

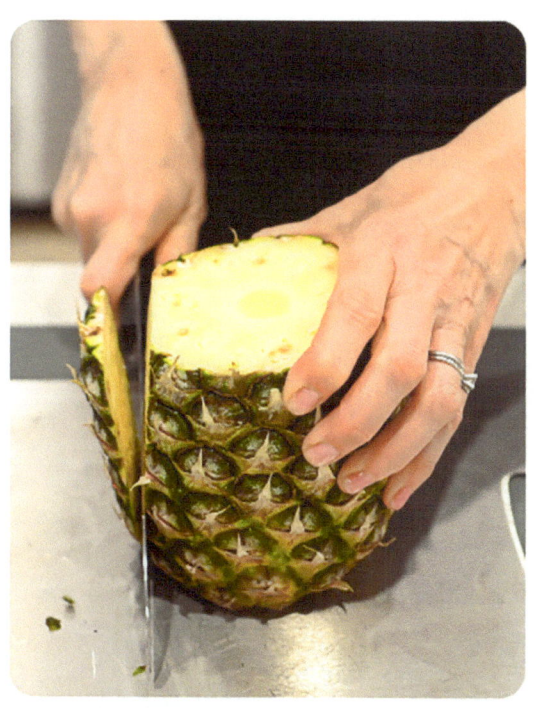

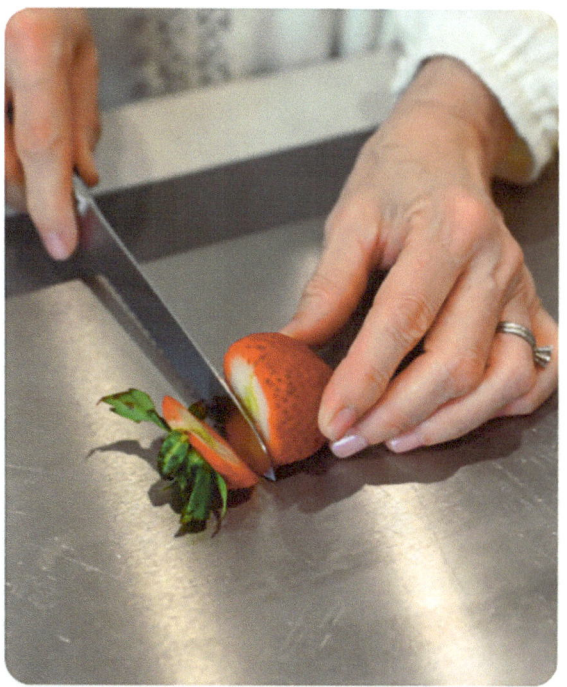

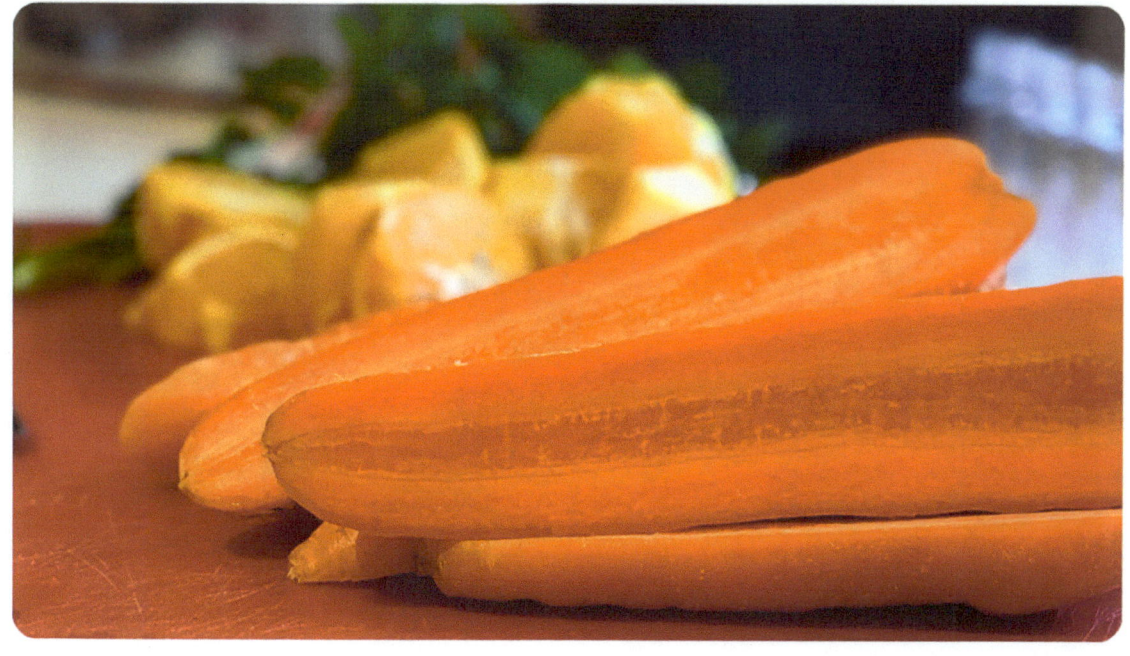

PHOTOGRAPHING
The Juicy Truth

Holly did all the shopping on a Thursday, visiting four different stores to gather the produce. She froze an entire case of bananas and stocked up on all the pantry staples & frozen fruit to prepare for the shoot. Friday, the day before the photoshoot, she spent 10 hours—start to finish, including cleanup—making all the juices, elixirs, sweet treats, and puddings.

Saturday, the day of the shoot, Holly had her hair and makeup done before everything kicked off at 2 p.m. During the 6-hour session, all the smoothies, açaí and smoothie bowls, and mocktails were made, juices were poured, and pictures were taken. After wrapping up and cleaning, Holly sent everyone home with plenty of delicious treats.

Behind every beautiful photo is a story of effort, intention, and heart. This shoot wasn't just about capturing images; it was about honoring every recipe, every moment, and every ounce of love poured into The Juicy Truth. Every item in the book was thoughtfully made and photographed; not just to look good, but to capture the joy and nourishment each one offers. A true labor of **LOVE**.

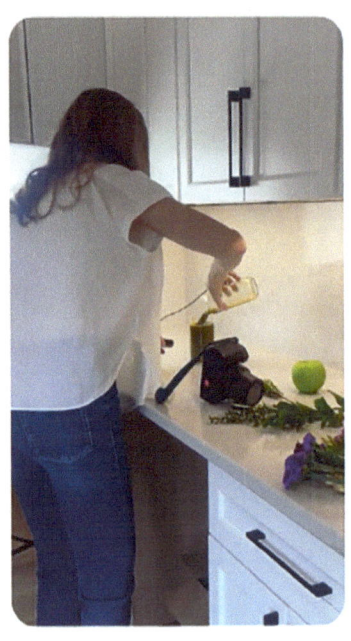 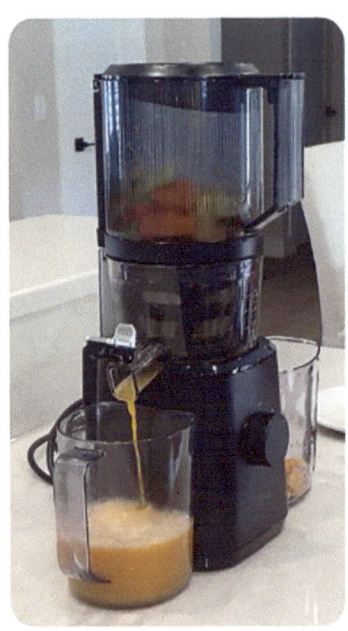 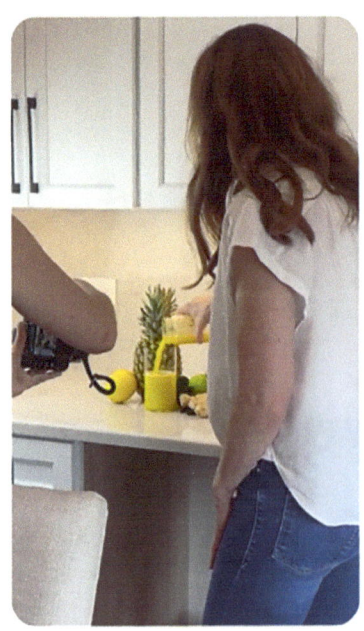

COLOR CODING MENU

The Little Apple™ Café menu was color coded to help customers find items they were looking for on the menu easily.

For example, **pineapple**paradise contains pineapple & mango and the finished product comes out yellow. While the zeus contains celery & kale and the finished product is a green juice. The **browns** contain cacao, chocolate protein, peanut butter, or almond butter. The red in the **super**detox is because the juice contains beets and comes out a deep red color.

This kept our menu fun and helped customers find items on our menu faster. The color coding only applied to the juice and smoothies. The rest of the menu we used green to match the cafés branding colors.

We organized the recipe book the similarly in hopes it would help you find what you are looking for easier. All recipes are alphabetized in their section, too.

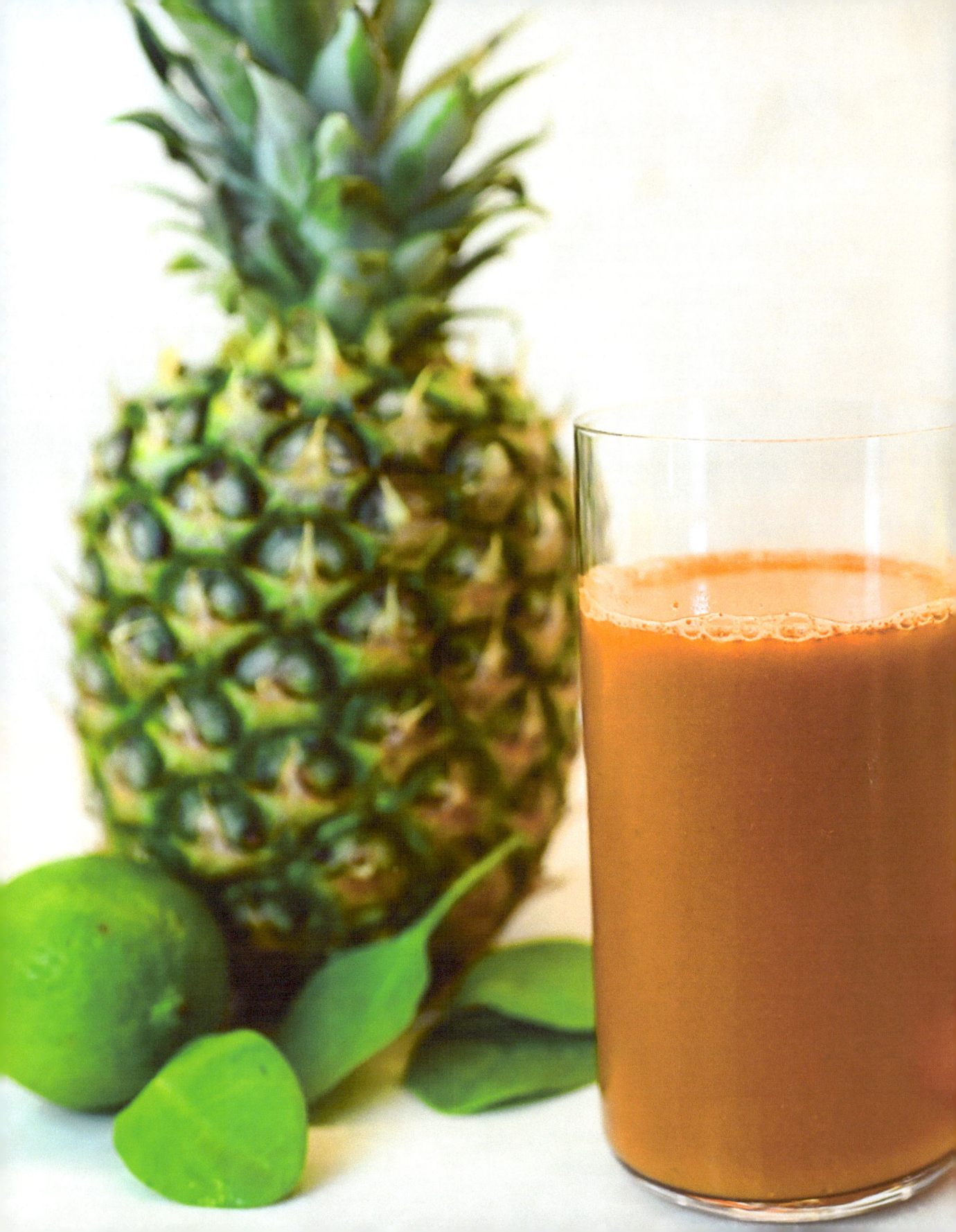

fresh pressed juice

At Home Juicer Recommendation:

Holly loves the Nama J2 Cold Press Juicer for juicing at home—it's hands-free, nutrient-preserving, and a serious time-saver.

Coming from commercial equipment, that's saying a lot. It's compact, easy to clean, and delivers incredible cold-pressed juice right in your kitchen.

This juicer can be purchased from **namawell.com**.

Use code **HOLLY10** at check out.

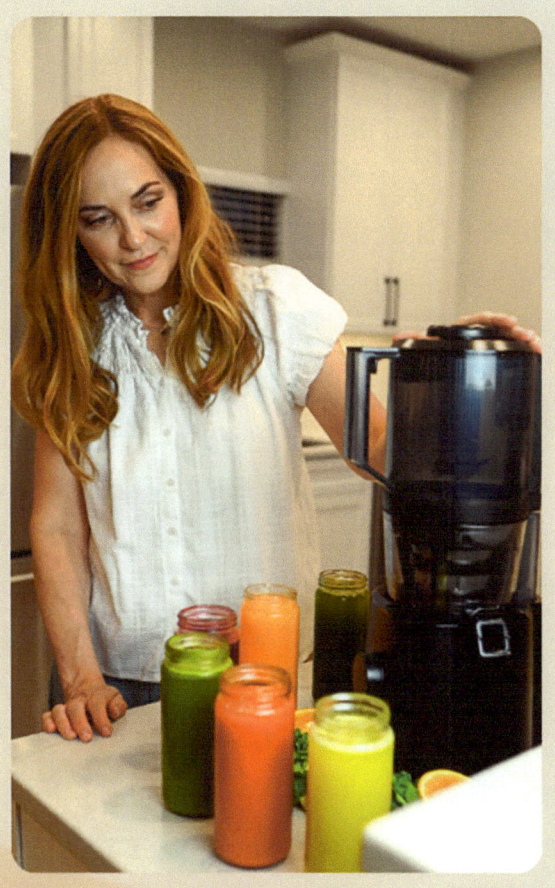

FRESH JUICE TIPS

Yield:
All juice recipes yield about 16 fluid oz. If your recipe falls short, you can always add more of an ingredient that produces a lot of juice (e.g., apple, carrot, cucumber).

Juicing Order:
When making multiple juices, start with the green juices first, then juice the other fruits/vegetables in order of color. Always juice the beets last to preserve the true colors of the other recipes. You can also run a small amount of water through the juicer between recipes to clean it.

Juicing Greens:
If your recipe includes kale, spinach, parsley, cilantro, mint, or ginger, put those items in the juicer first. If your juicer requires you to push ingredients through individually, alternate the greens with juicier items.

Cutting Produce:
For best results, cut the fruits and vegetables into smaller pieces depending on your juicer. Large commercial juicers may allow you to insert a whole carrot, while home juicers typically require smaller pieces.

Granny Smith Apples:
Use Granny Smith apples, as they contain less sugar and are crisp, juicy, and tart, giving your juice a nice flavor. Cut the apples into quarters and remove the core and seeds.

Ginger:

 A "knob" of ginger is about 1 inch. Since ginger can vary in spiciness, do a taste test and adjust the amount to your liking.

Citrus:

Peel off all citrus fruits before juicing.

Storage:

Fresh-pressed juice can be stored in a tightly sealed container (preferably glass) for a maximum of 3-4 days. For best results, fill the container to the top to minimize air exposure. Shake well before drinking.

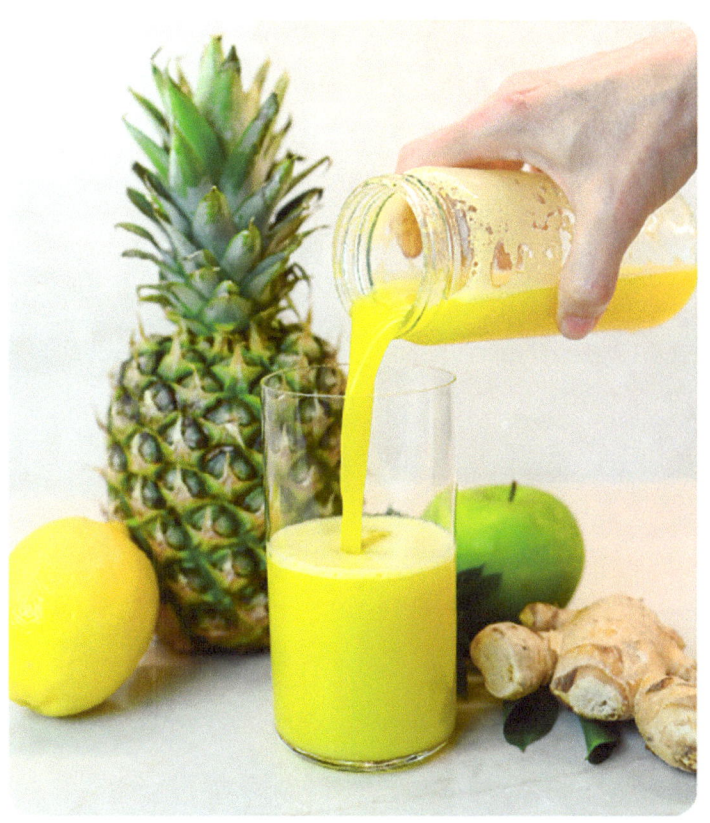

Freezing Juice Instructions:

Juices can be frozen—just pour into a freezer-safe container and leave some space at the top to allow for expansion. Use within 3–4 months. To defrost, transfer to the fridge or place the container in cold water to speed up the process. Shake well before drinking.

beeting**heart**

Ingredients

- 1 medium beet (4 ounces)
- 2 pineapple spears (4 ounces)
- 3 medium strawberries (2 ounces)
- 1 apple (2 ounces)
- 1 knob of ginger (1 ounce)
- 1 orange (3 ounces)

This juice recipe was a secret recipe that was never on the menu and was only shared with staff.

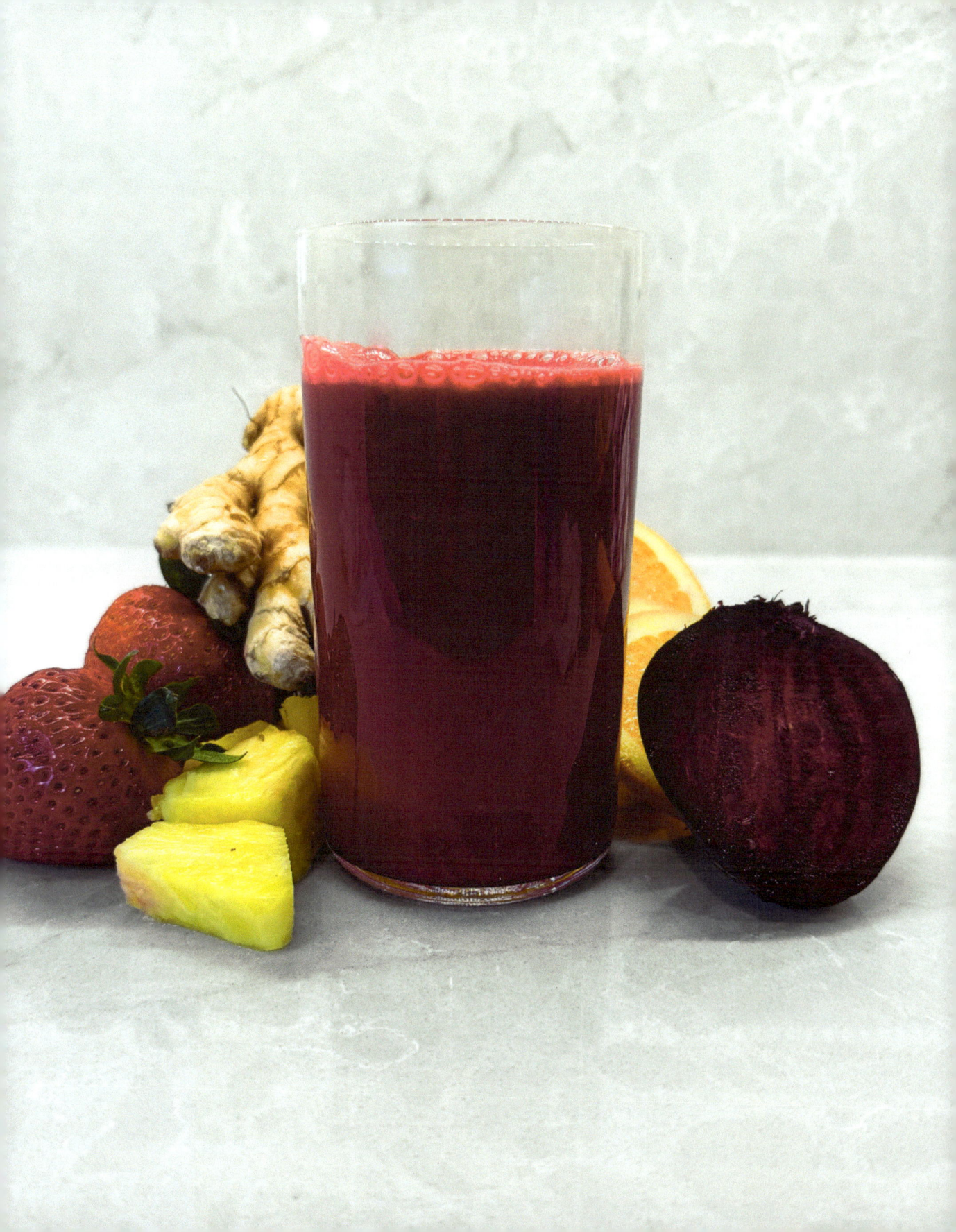

bodyelectric

Ingredients

- 3 medium carrots (7 ounces)
- 2 pineapple spears (6 ounces)
- 4 handfuls of spinach (2 ounces)
- 1 lime (1 ounce)

TIP

 For best results, put spinach in first, then lime, pineapple, and carrots.

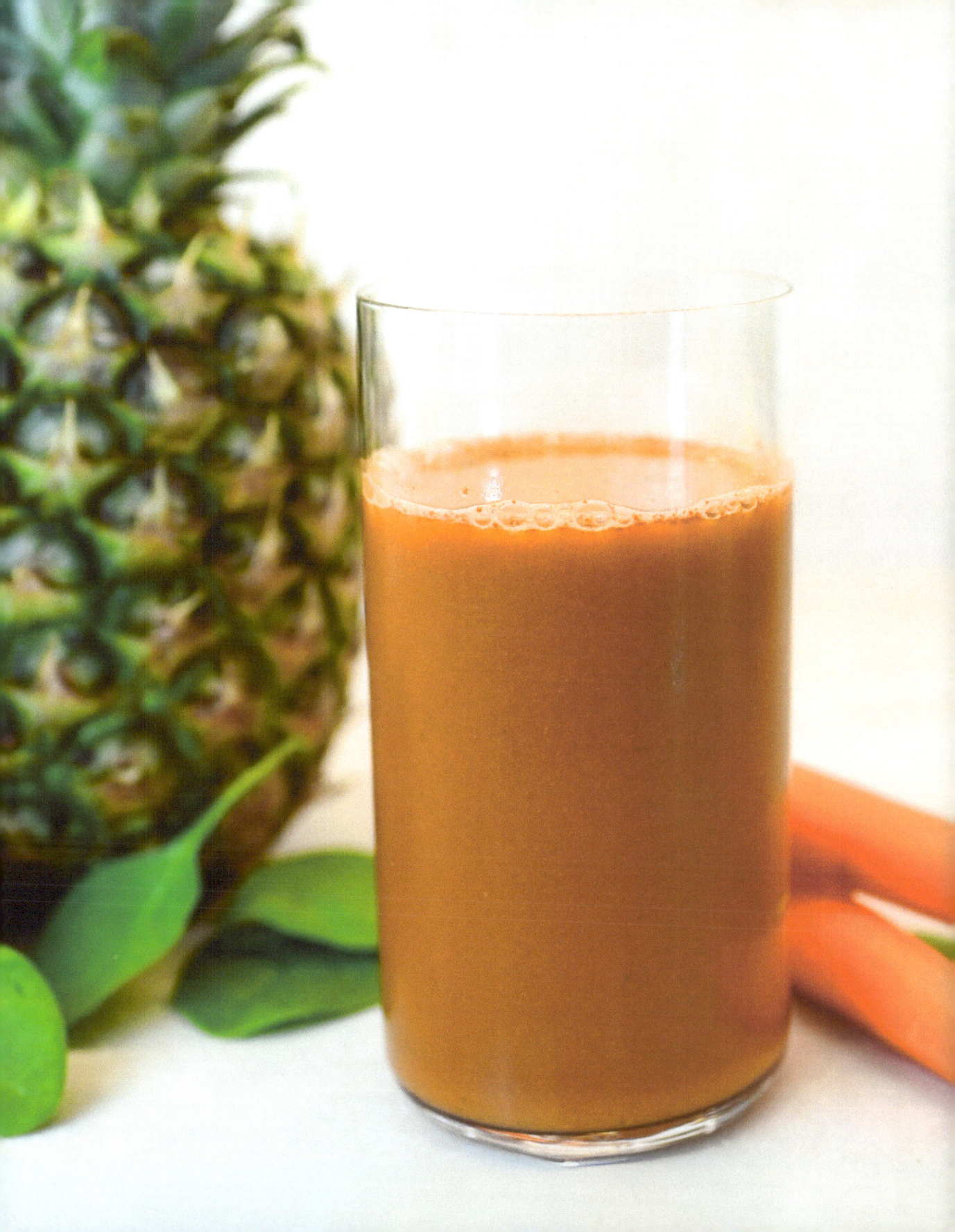

goldenglow

juice

Ingredients

- 2 apples (5 ounces)
- 4 medium carrots (9 ounces)
- 1 lemon (1 ounce)
- 1 knob of ginger (1 ounce)

The goldenglow was the #1 juice of all time. One time we had someone order 14 bottles at once!

Pairs well with:

- 1 pineapple spear for a more filling sweet taste
- 1 knob (about 1 inch) of turmeric (or to taste)

TIP

 For best results, add ginger, lemon, carrot, and then apple.

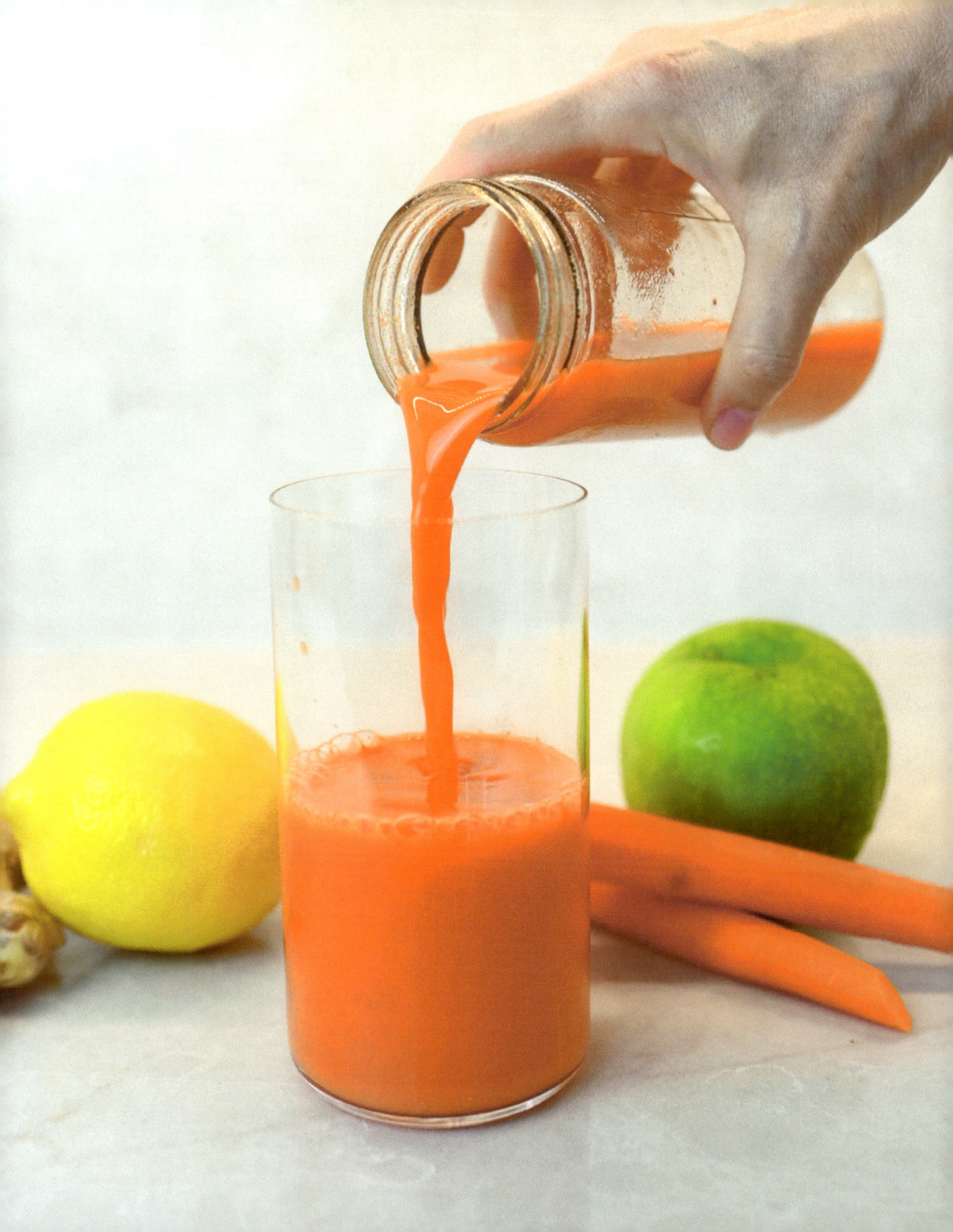

greenlemonade

The greenlemonade was the #1 selling green juice. Even kids love this one!

Ingredients

- 2 apples (5 ounces)
- 1 medium cucumber (8 ounces)
- 2-3 kale leaves (2 ounces)
- 1 lemon (1 ounce)

Pairs well with:

- 1 knob of ginger for a little zing

TIP

 For best results, put the kale leaves in first, followed by lemon, cucumber, and apples.

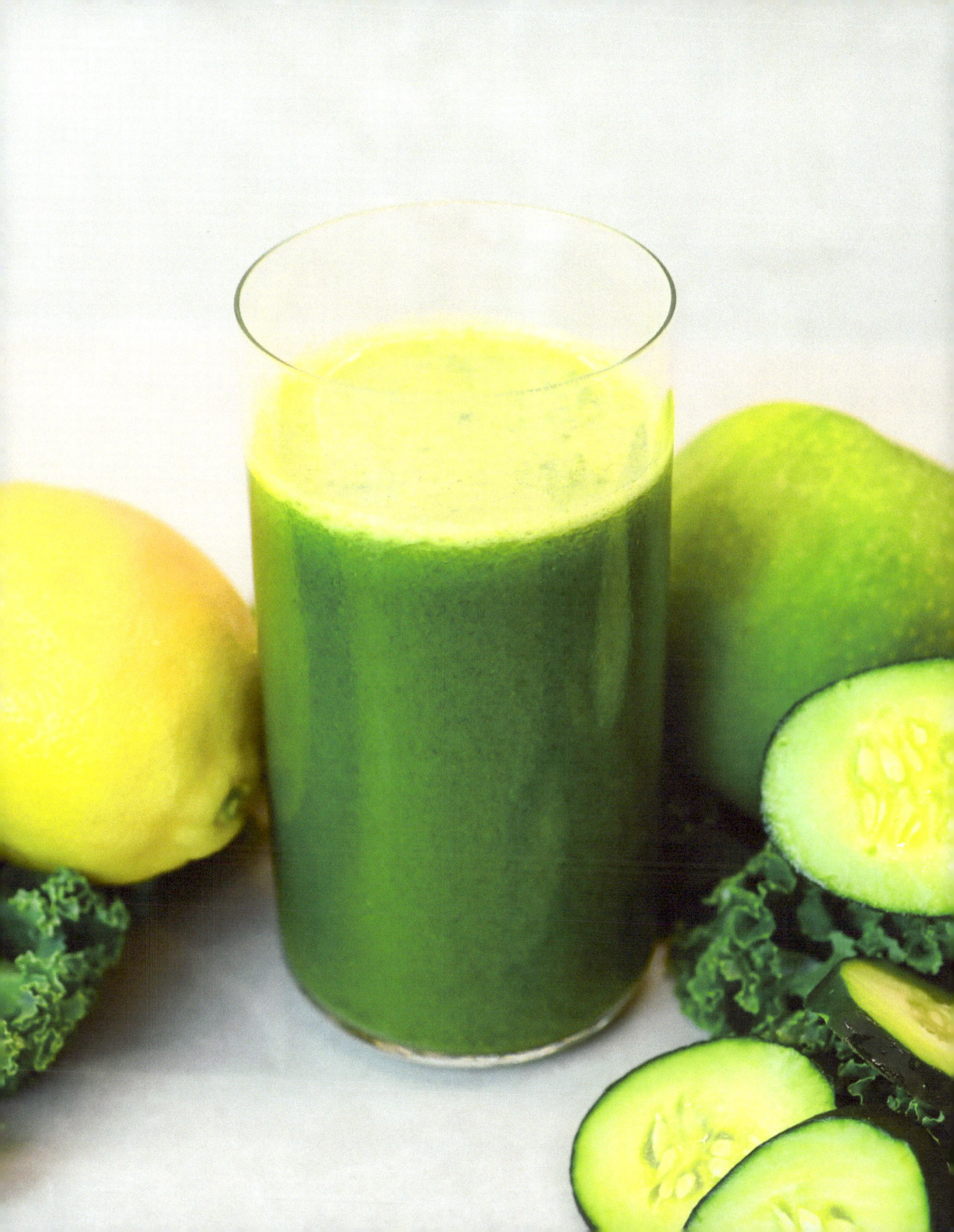

immunity

juice

Ingredients

- 4 medium carrots (8 ounces)
- 2 large oranges (6 ounces)
- large handful of mint (1 ounce)
- large handful of parsley (1 ounce)

TIP

 For best results, put mint & parsley in first, then oranges and carrots.

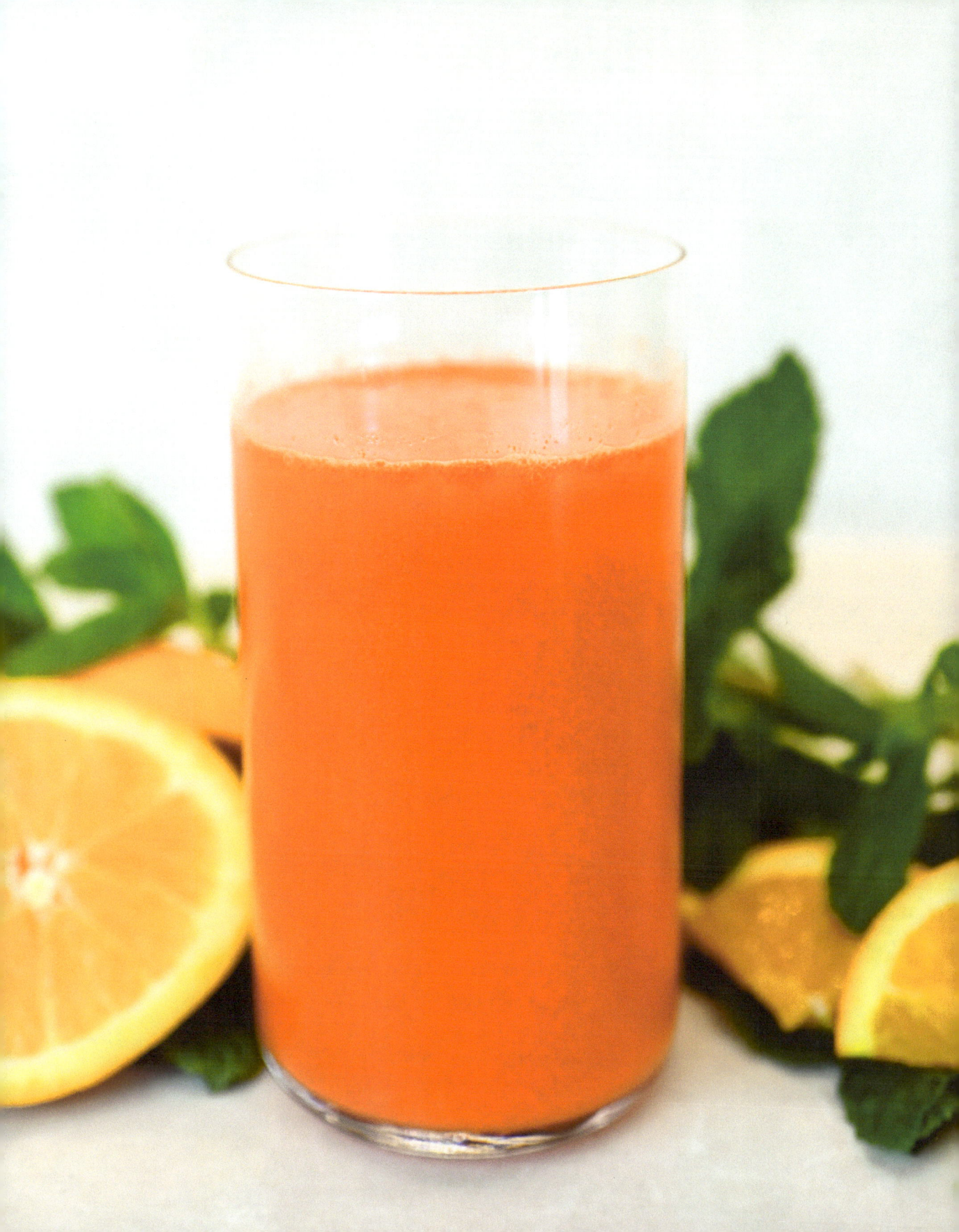

littlegreenapple

Ingredients

- 5 celery stalks (5 ounces)
- 2 apples (5 ounces)
- 2 pineapple spears (4 ounces)
- 4 handfuls of spinach (1 ounce)
- 1 lime (1 ounce)
- handful of mint (6 mint leaves)

TIP

 For best results, add spinach and mint in first, followed by pineapple, celery, and apples.

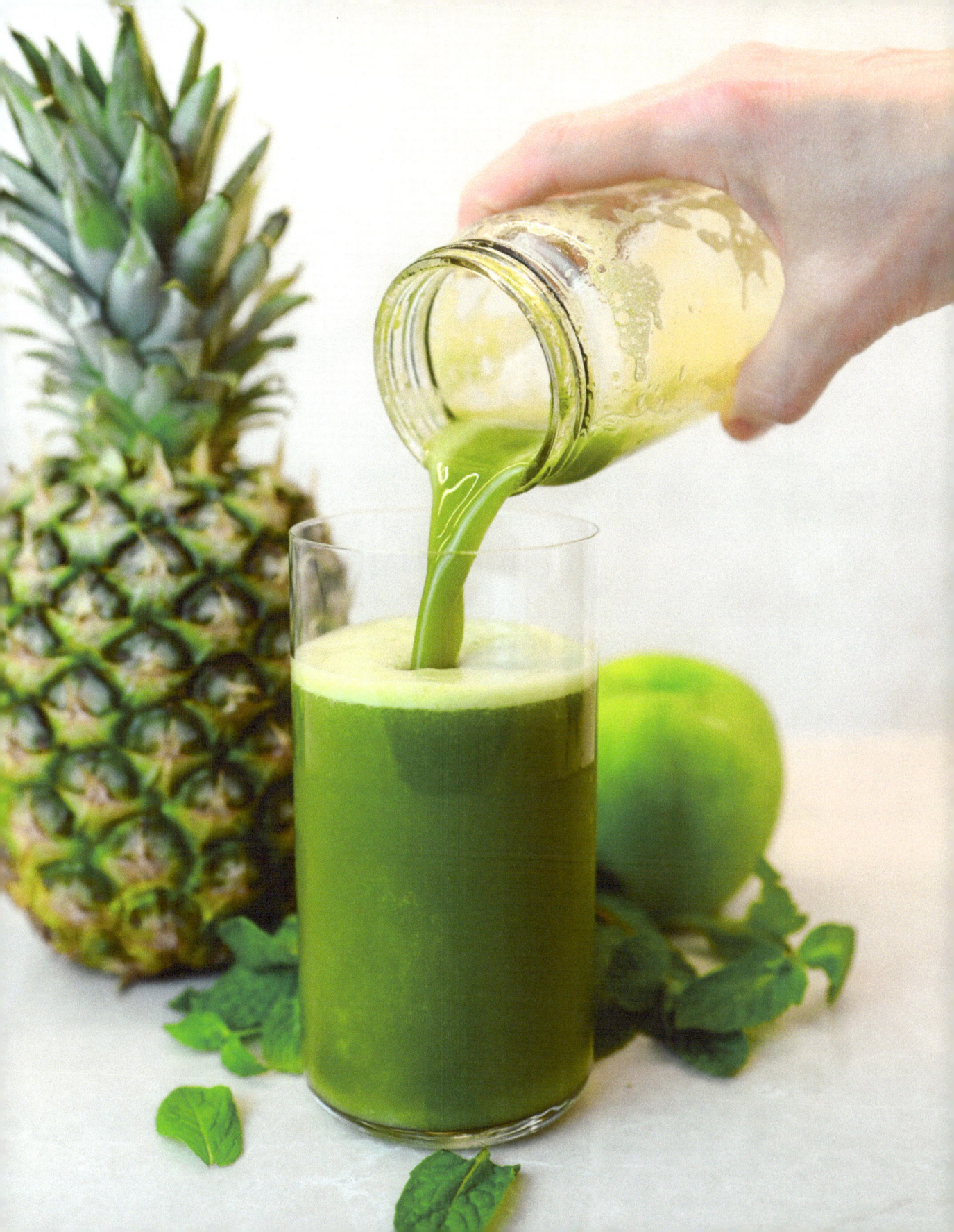

malibu

juice

Ingredients

- 2 apples (6 ounces)
- 3 pineapple spears (7 ounces)
- 1 lemon (2 ounces)
- 1 knob ginger (1 ounce)
- handful of mint (6 mint leaves)

The malibu was used to make cocktails at the café. We used it in our housemade margaritas.

TIPS

 For best results, put ginger and mint in first, followed by lemon, pineapple and apple.

 Add 2 ounces of malibu juice to your favorite margarita on the rocks.

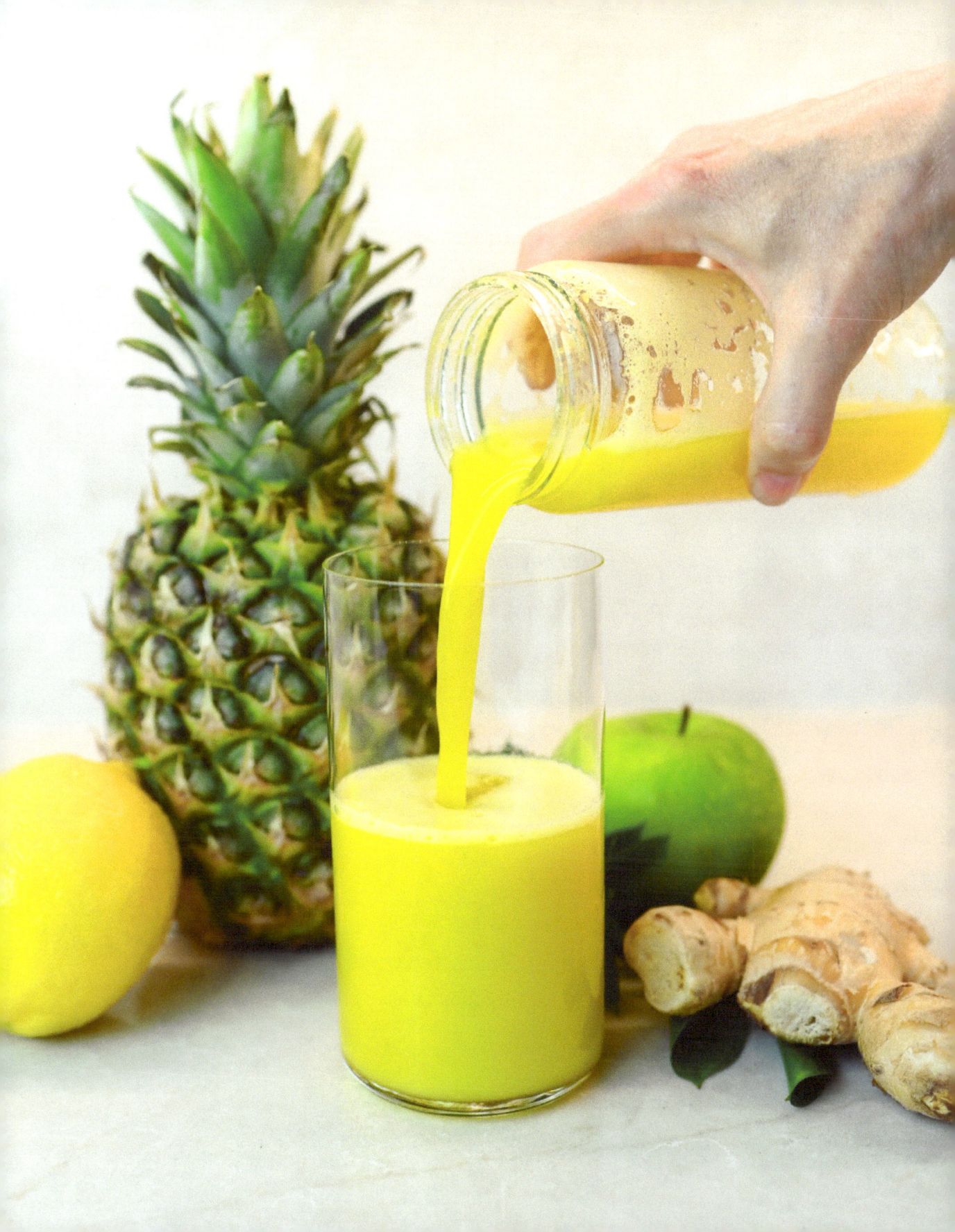

meangreen

juice

Ingredients

- 1 small cucumber (4 ounces)
- 5 celery stalkers (5 ounces)
- 4 handfuls of spinach (2 ounces)
- 2 apples (5 ounces)

 Time Saver:

Purchase triple-washed spinach directly from the store to save prep time.

TIP

 For best results, add your spinach in first, followed by celery, cucumber, and then apples.

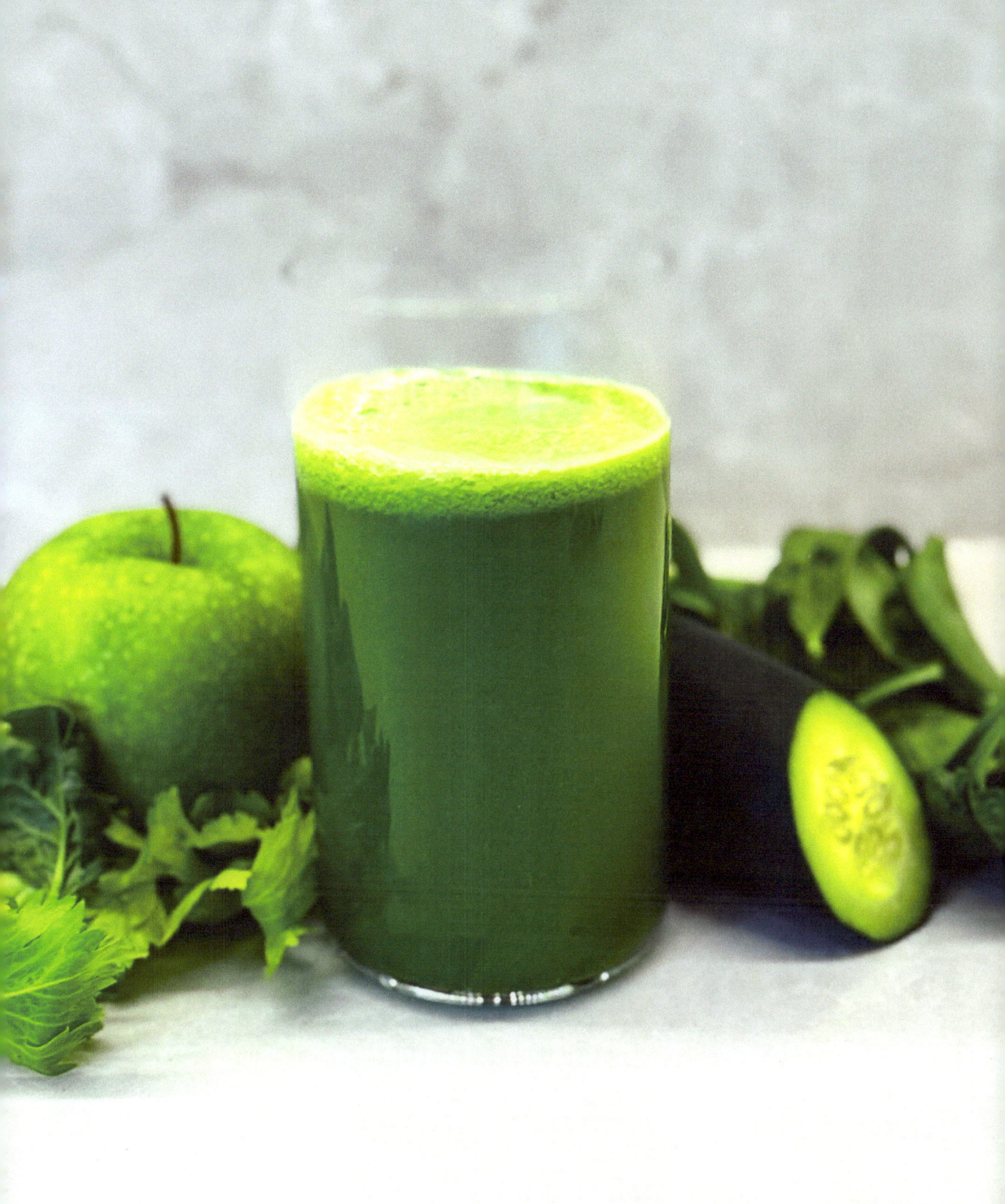

recovery

Ingredients

- 3 kale leaves (2 ounces)
- handful of cilantro (2 ounces)
- 4 handfuls of spinach (2 ounces)
- 5-6 carrots (for remaining 10 ounces)

TIP

 For best results, alternate carrots in between kale, cilantro, and spinach.

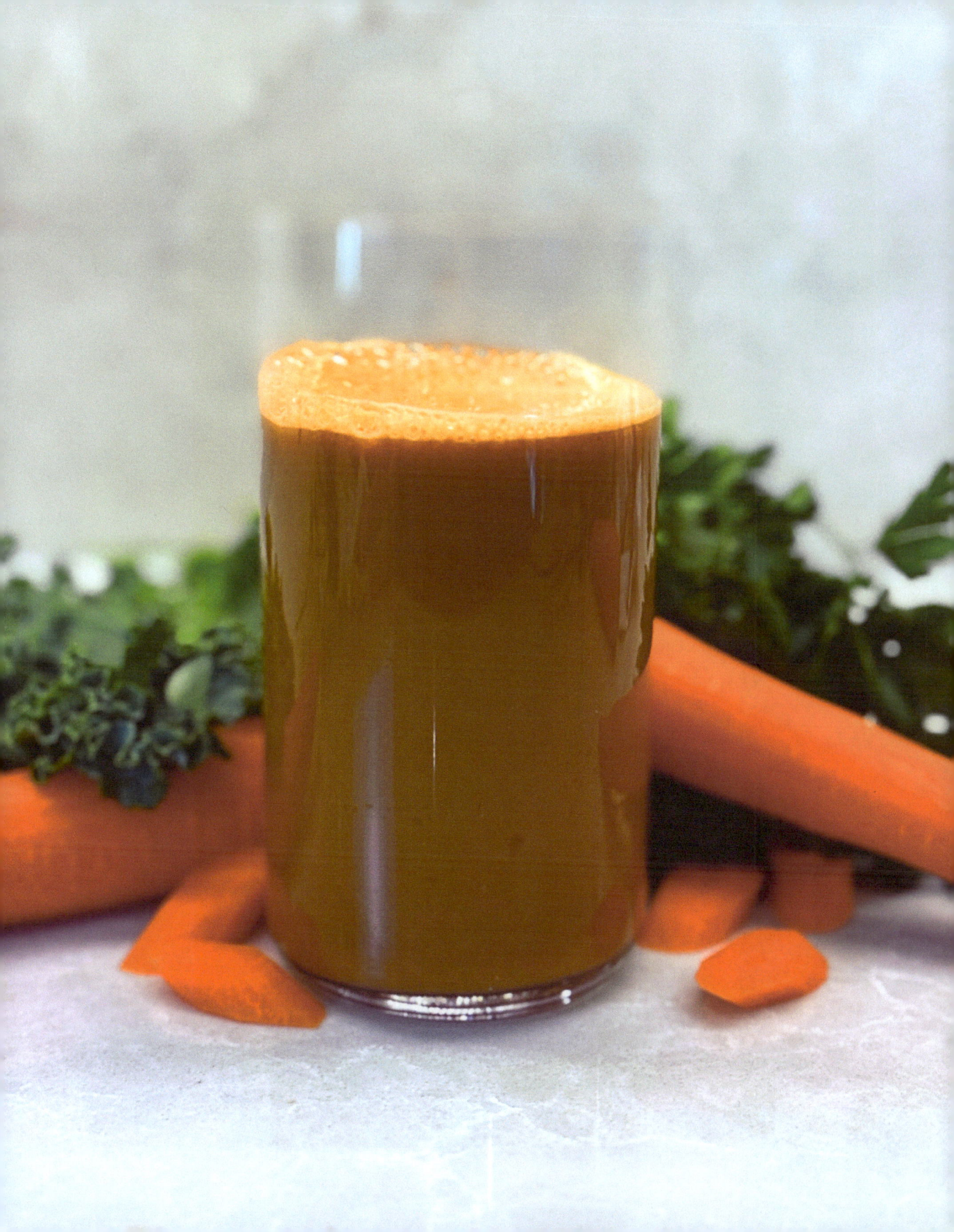

skinnygreens

Ingredients

- 5 celery stalks (7 ounces)
- 1 small cucumber (6 ounces)
- 2 kale leaves (1 ounce)
- handful of parsley (1 ounce)
- 1 lemon (1 ounce)

TIP

 For best results, add parsley and kale in first, followed by lemon, celery, and cucumber.

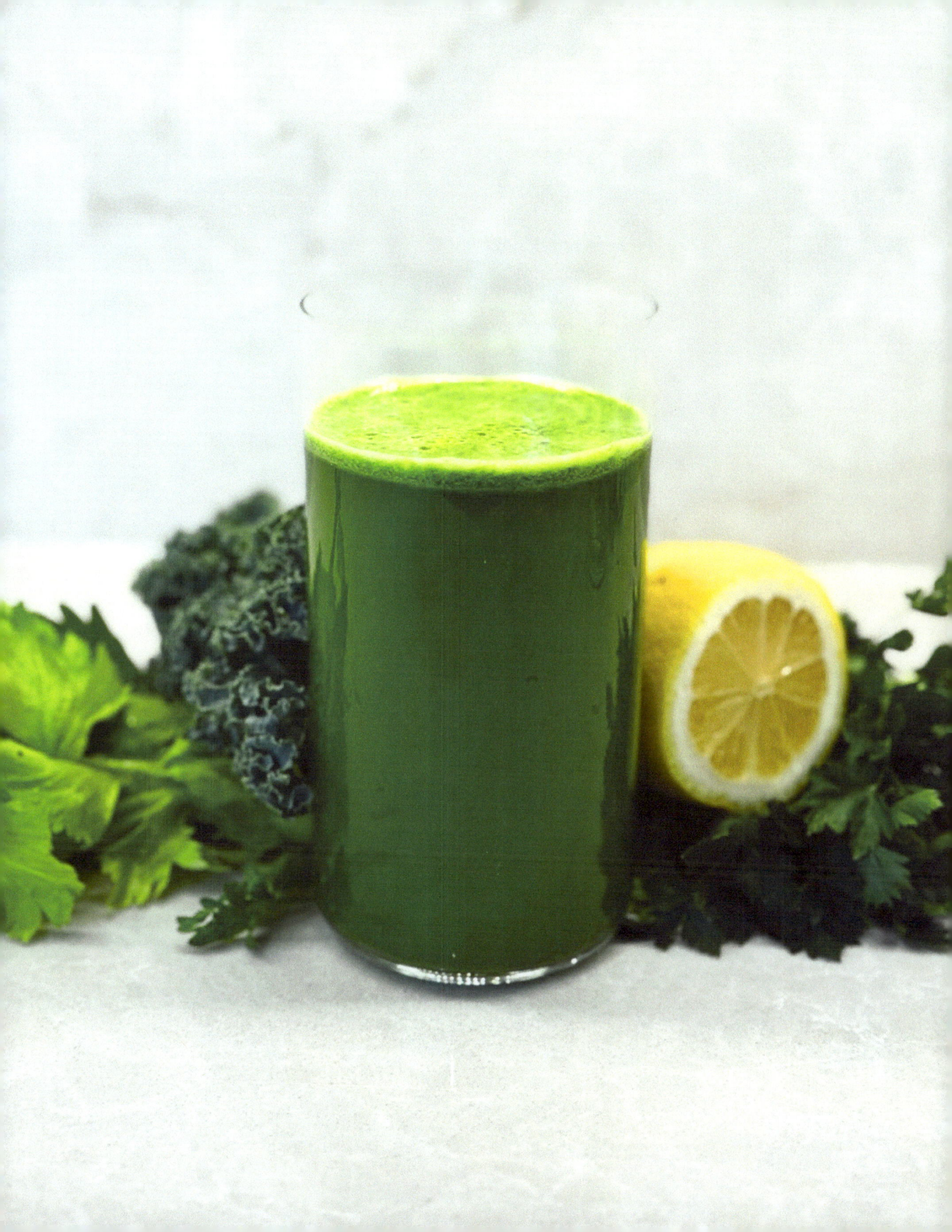

super**detox**

Ingredients

- 2 apples (5 ounces)
- 2 medium carrots (5 ounces)
- 1 medium red beet (5 ounces)
- 1 lemon (1 ounce)

Pairs well with:

- 1 knob of ginger (or to taste) for a little zing
- 1 pineapple spear for a more filling sweet taste

TIP

 For best results, add beets first, followed by lemon, carrots, and then apples.

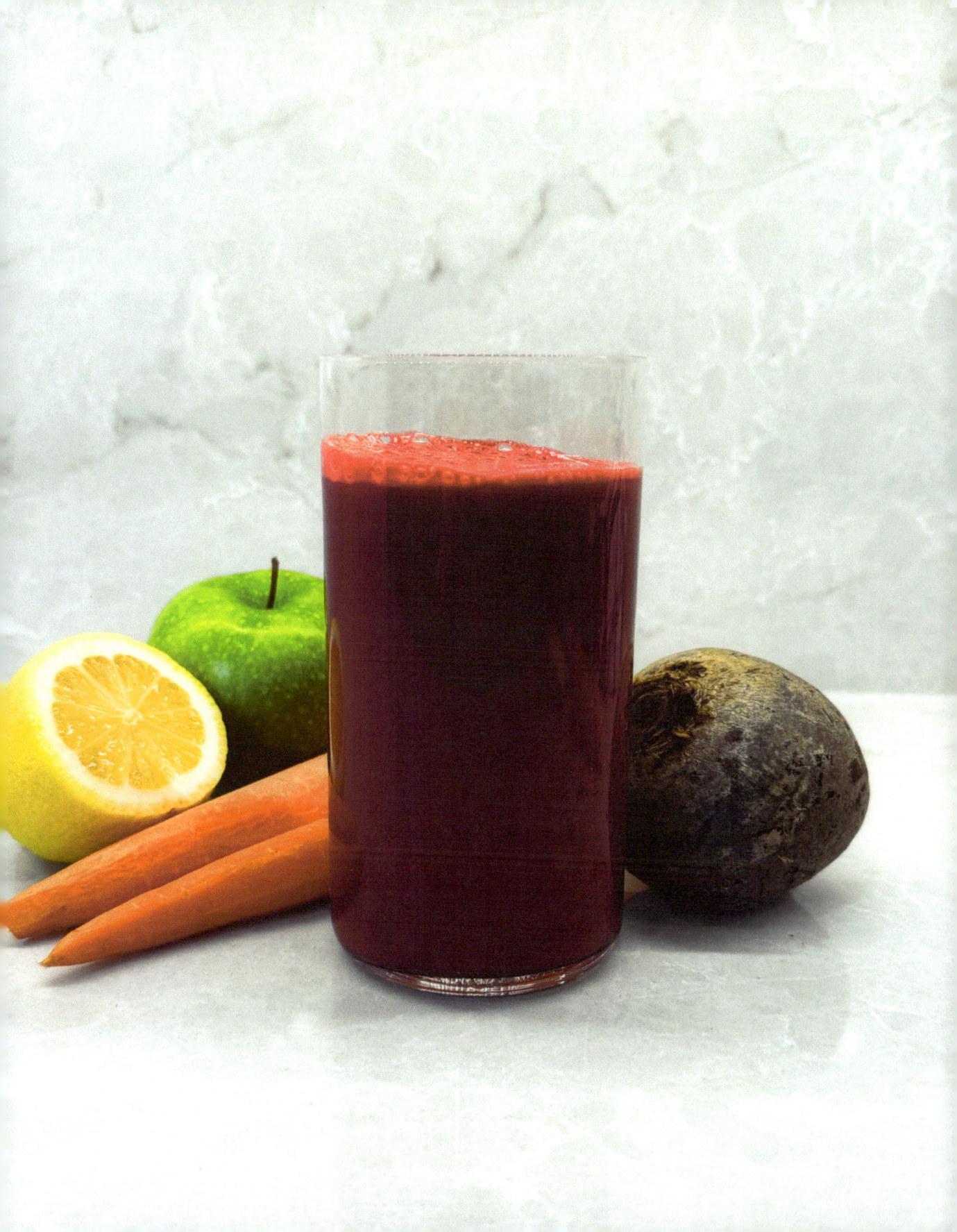

zeus

juice

Ingredients

- 2 apples (5 ounces)
- 5 celery stalks (7 ounces)
- 2-3 kale leaves (2 ounces)
- 1 knob of ginger (2 ounces)

Pairs well with:

- 1 lemon for a refreshing twist
- 1 pineapple spear for a more filling sweet taste

TIP

 For best results, put the ginger and kale in the juicer first, followed by the celery and apples.

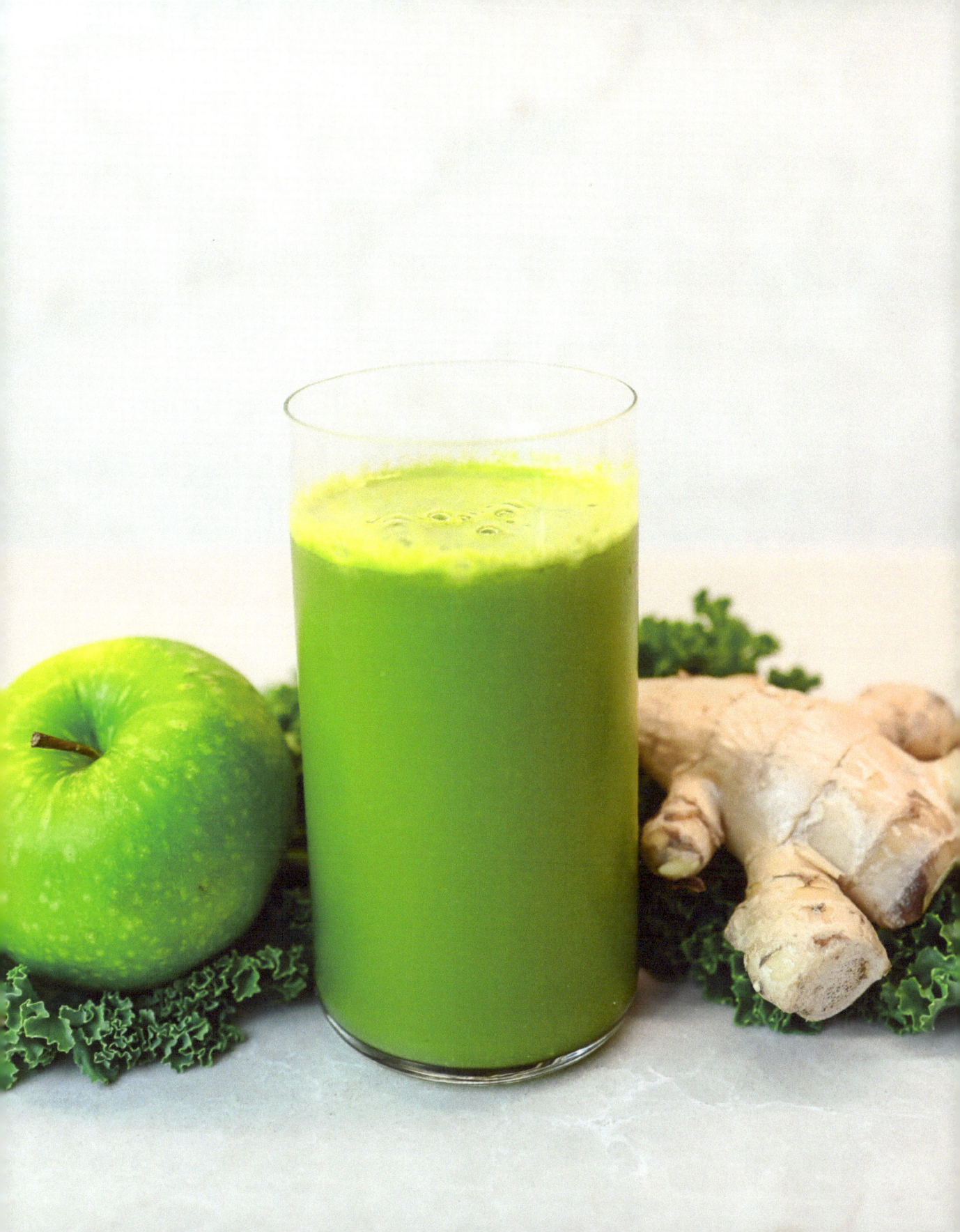

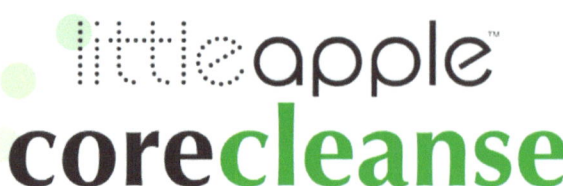

littleapple™
corecleanse

This **3-day corecleanse** was a big hit at the cafe. If done correctly by the customer, the corecleanse would detox them from sugar, caffeine, and also serve as a mini reset to cleanse the pallet from junk food.

For the best results, we recommend the juicing schedule provided. The corecleanse is designed to provide a **refreshing reset**, offering a balanced combination of fruits and vegetables to support your body's natural processes. Packed with essential nutrients, this cleanse **helps replenish your body and promote hydration**.

After completing the cleanse, you may feel refreshed, lighter, and experience improved energy levels.

On the next few pages, you'll find the recipes and instructions to our infamous corecleanse. Now you can make your own cleanse at home!

TIPS

❋ Each core cleanse juice recipe makes 16 fluid ounce per juice.

❋ If you want to cleanse more than one day, multiply each recipe by the amount of days. For a 3-day juice cleanse, you need 48 fluid ounce of each juice.

little apple™
corecleanse

For the best results, we recommend following this juicing schedule:

1 ravishingruby   **7/9am**

Rich in nutrients and antioxidants, this Beet, Carrot, and Apple juice is a refreshing blend may help to support the body's natural detox pathways and promote overall wellness.

2 elixir   **Before 12pm**

Your choice of 2oz Aloe or Chlorophyl elixir

3 chinatown80   **11am/12pm**

Hydrate and refresh with this zesty blend of Pomegranate, Orange, Coconut Water, Lime, Ginger, and Beet. Rich in antioxidants and naturally hydrating, which may help to support their body's natural detox and feel their best.

4 elfuego   **1/2pm**

Grapefruit Juice, Orange Juice, Cayenne. Enjoy the fat-burning magic of Cayenne, with all the Vitamin C you ever wanted. It's sinfully delicious.

5 masterblaster   **3/4pm**

Made with Lemon, Ginger, Filtered Water, and a hint of Maple Syrup, this refreshing blend supports hydration, digestion, and immune wellness—perfect for a natural reset.

6 thehulk   **5/6pm**

Celery, Cucumber, Spirulina, Flax Oil, Himalayan Salt. One of our greenest juices, thehulk literally packs a punch. A super immune booster!

7 dr.normselixir   **7/8pm**

Celery, Carrot, Spinach, Parsley. Dr Norman Walker, the inventor of the cold pressed juice, drank this juice every day!

Remember to drink plenty of water and if you need something warm try some decaf tea.

ravishingruby

corecleanse juice

Ingredients

- 2 apples (6 ounces)
- 3 medium carrots (6 ounces)
- 1 medium red beet (4 ounces)

TIP

 For best results, add beet first, followed by carrots and apples.

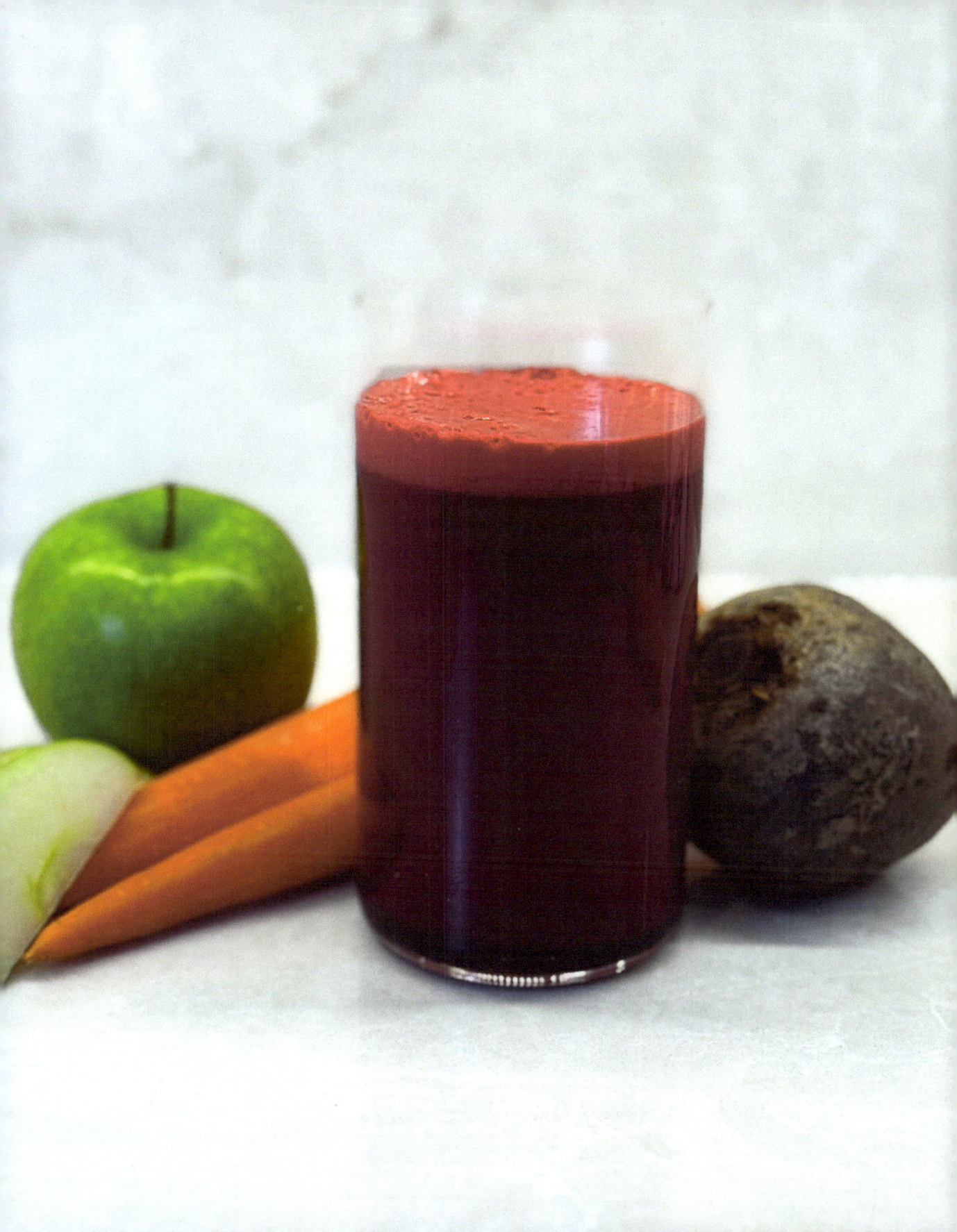

chlorophyl**shot**

corecleanse juice

Ingredients

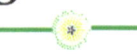

- ¼ teaspoon of chlorella powder
- 2 ounces of filtered water

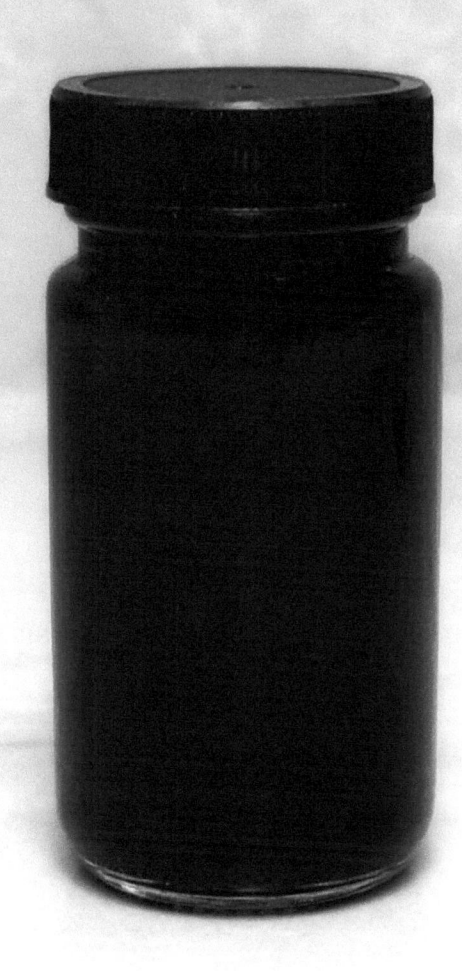

3

chinatown80

Ingredients

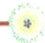

- 2 oranges (6 ounces)
- 1 pomegranate (3 ounces)
- 3 ounces of coconut water
- 1 red beet (2 ounces)
- 1 knob of ginger (1 ounce)
- 1 lime (1 ounce)

 Time Saver:

Purchase pomegranate concentrate from store. This is especially helpful if pomegranates are not in season.

TIP

 For best results, put beet and ginger in first, followed by pomegranate seeds, lime, and then orange. When finished juicing, add coconut water of your choice.

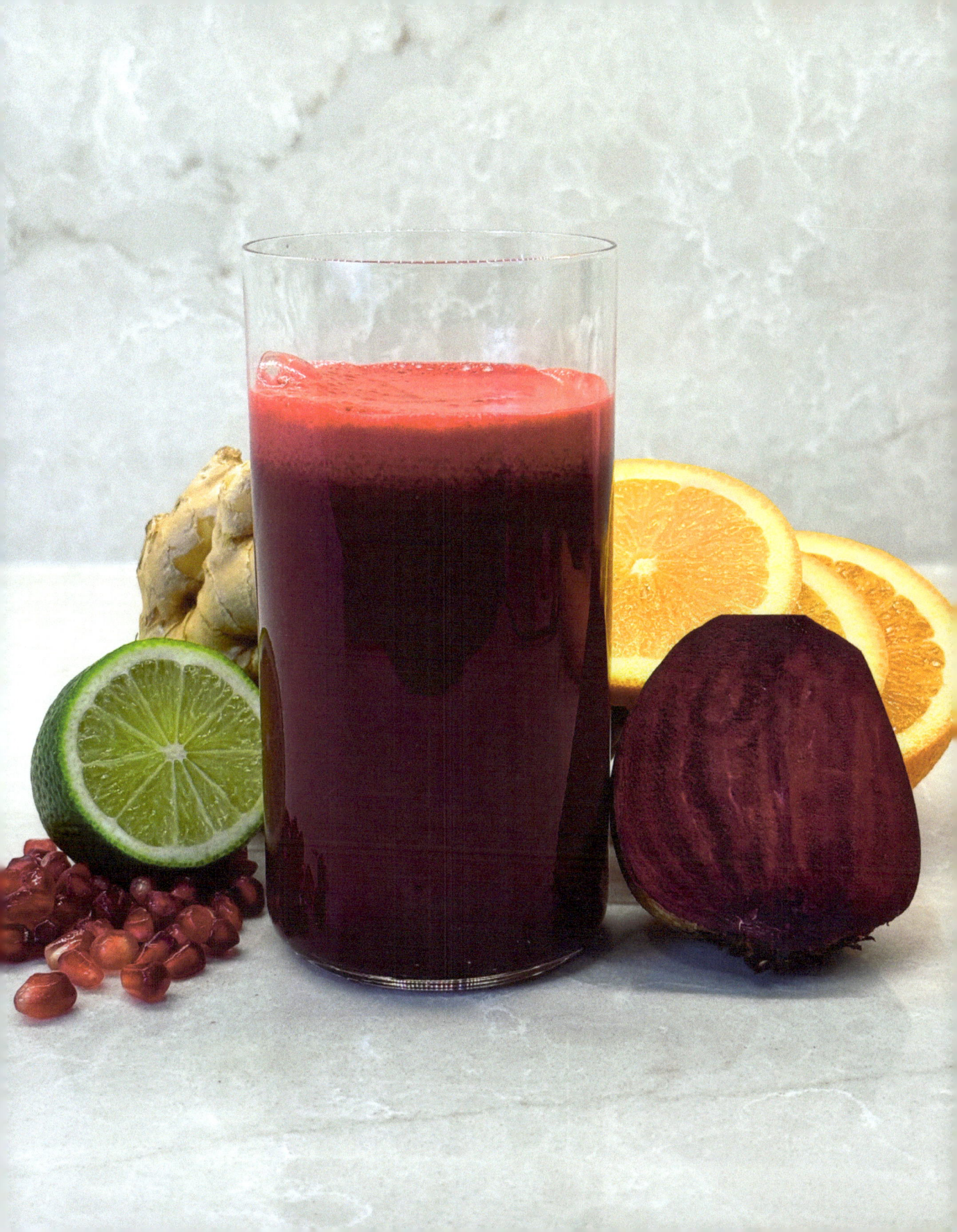

4

elfuego

corecleanse juice

Ingredients

- 2-3 oranges (8 ounces)
- 2 grapefruits (8 ounces)
- ¼ teaspoon of cayenne extract

elfuego was the most LOVED juice from the corecleanse.

TIP

 Juice oranges first, then grapefruit. Once mixed, add cayenne extract and stir.

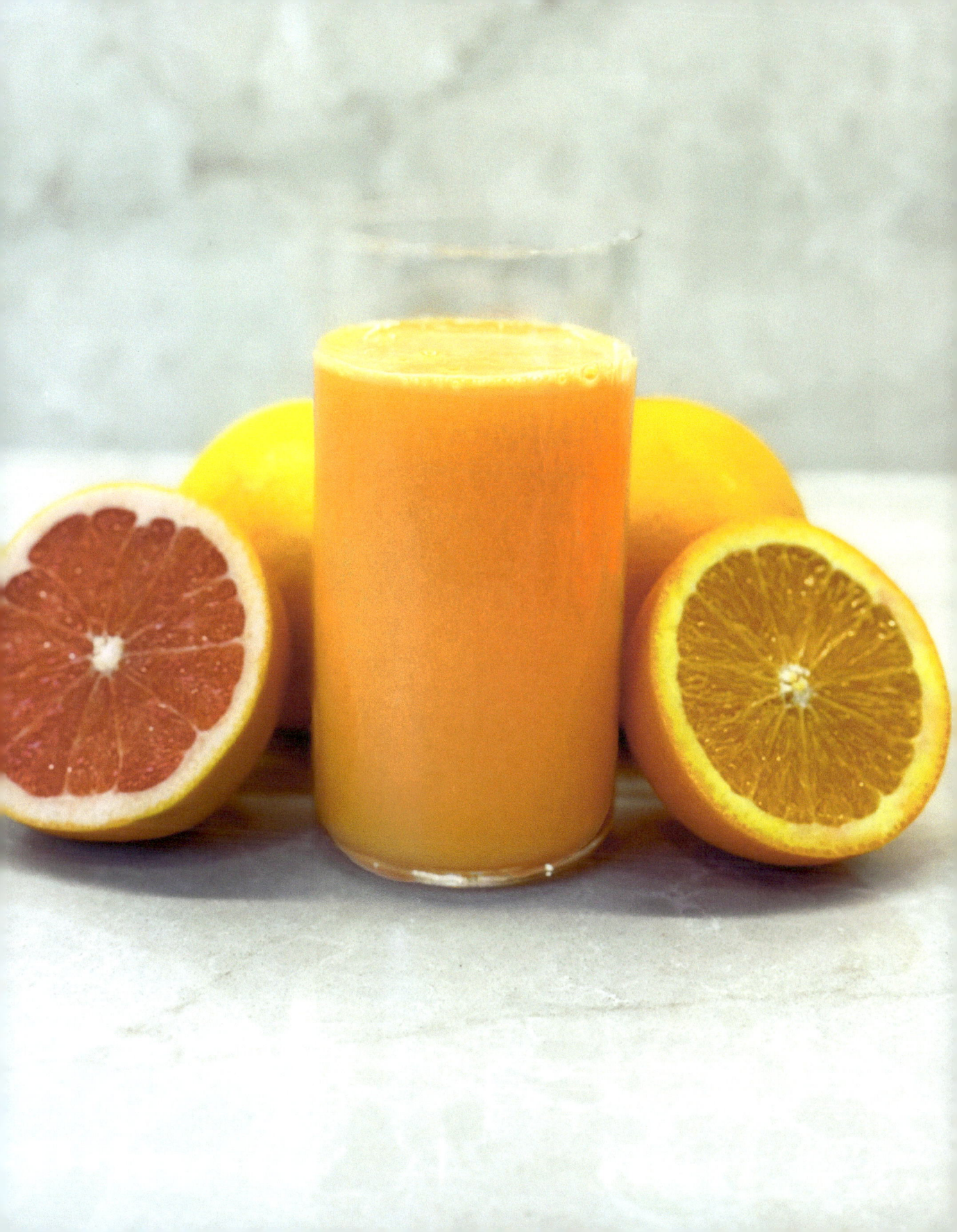

5

master**blaster**

Ingredients

- 3 lemons (5 ounces)
- 3 knobs of ginger (2 ounces)
- 8 ounces of filtered water
- 1 ounce maple syrup
- ¼ teaspoon cayenne extract

TIP

 Juice ginger first, then lemons. Then add water, maple syrup, and cayenne extract. Mix well.

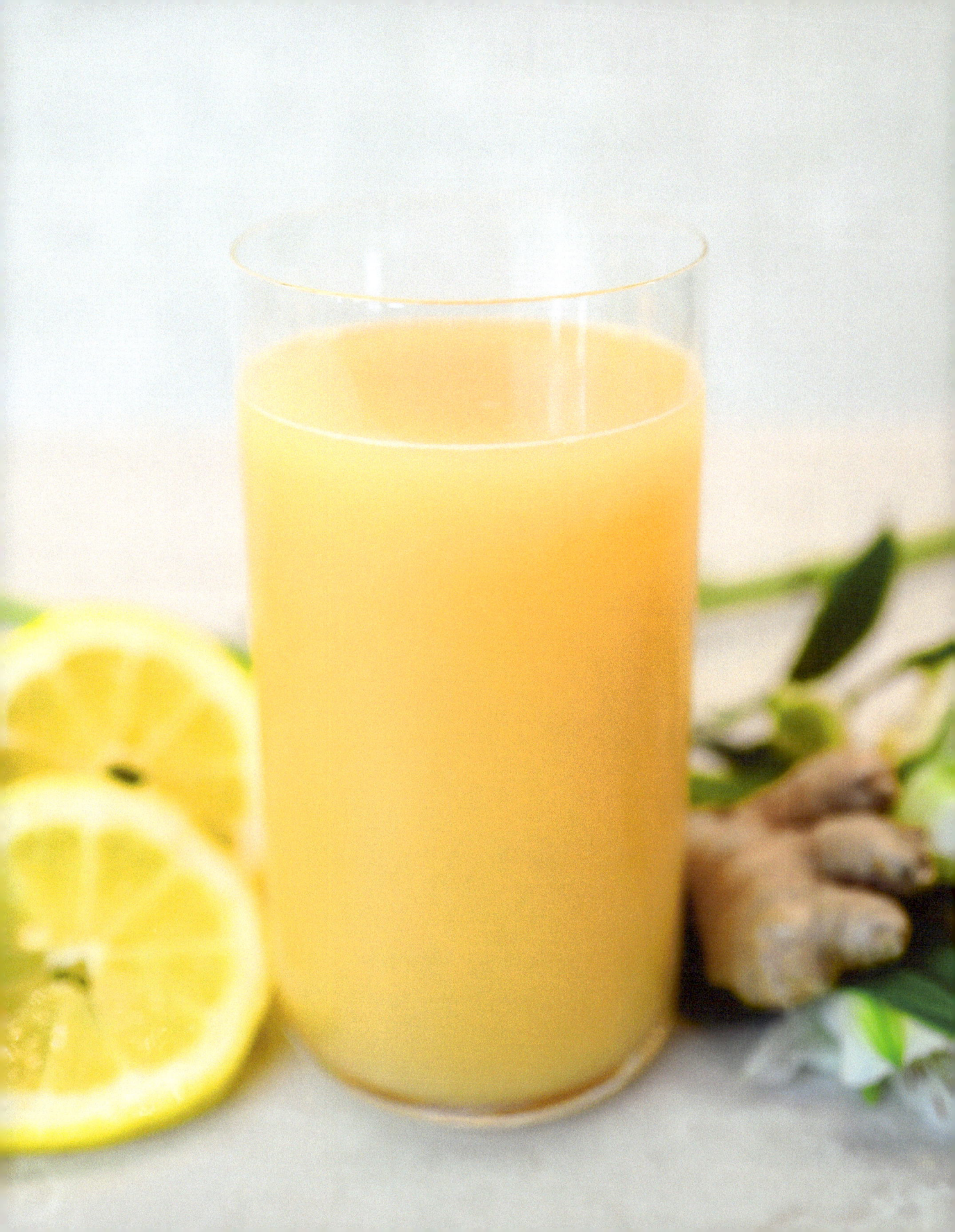

6

thehulk

Ingredients

- 1 medium cucumber (7 ounces)
- 5 celery stalks (6 ounces)
- 2-3 kale leaves (2 ounces)
- 1 ounce flax seed oil
- ¼ teaspoon spirulina
- ¼ teaspoon Himalayan salt

TIP

When juicing, alternate kale and celery, then finish with cucumber. Once completed, add flax seed oil, spirulina, and Himalayan salt. Mix well.

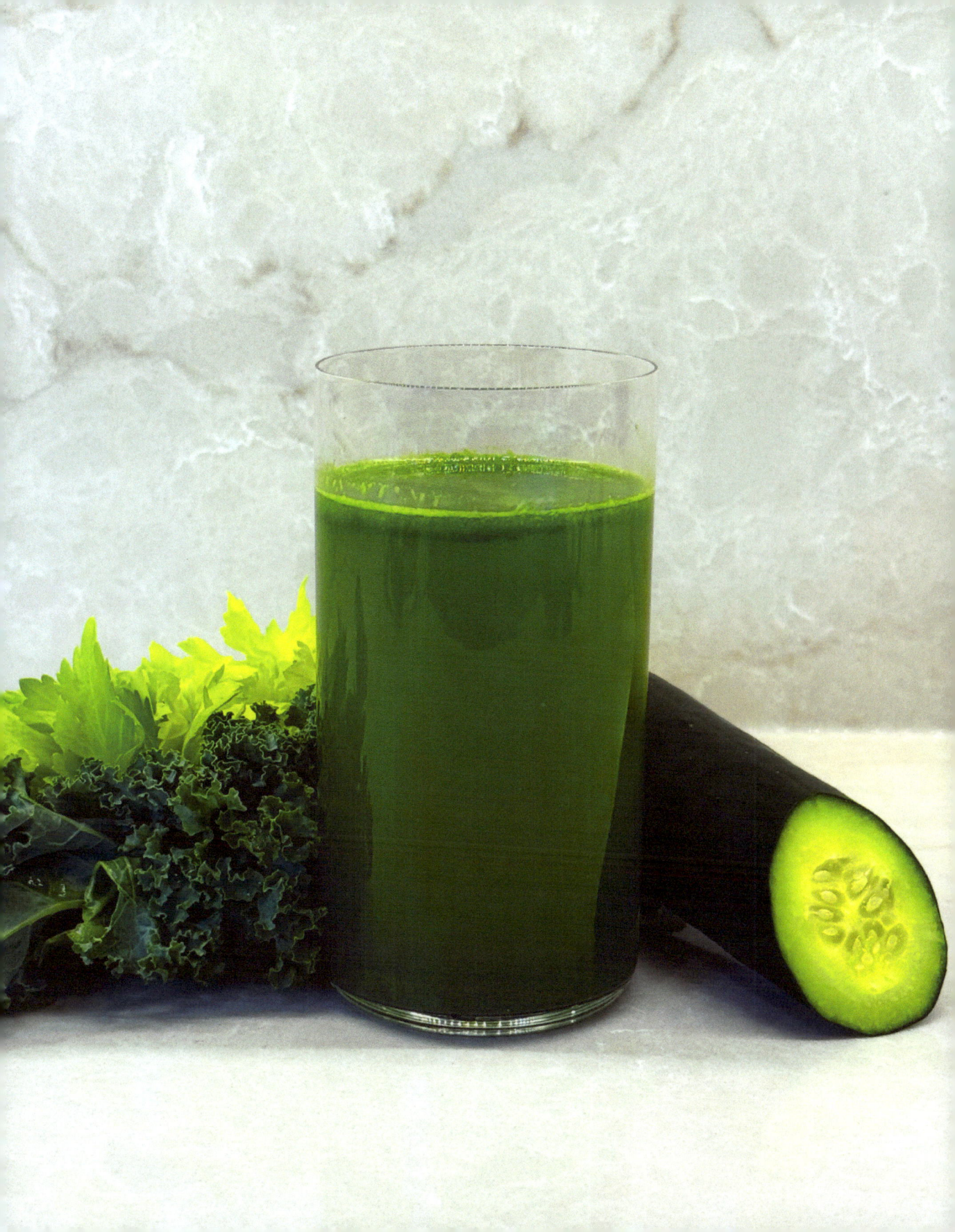

dr.normselixir

corecleanse juice

Ingredients

- 3 carrots (7 ounces)
- 5 celery stalks (6 ounces)
- 4 handfuls of spinach (2 ounces)
- handful of parsley (1 ounce)

TIP

 Juice parsley and spinach, alternating with celery, and finish with carrots.

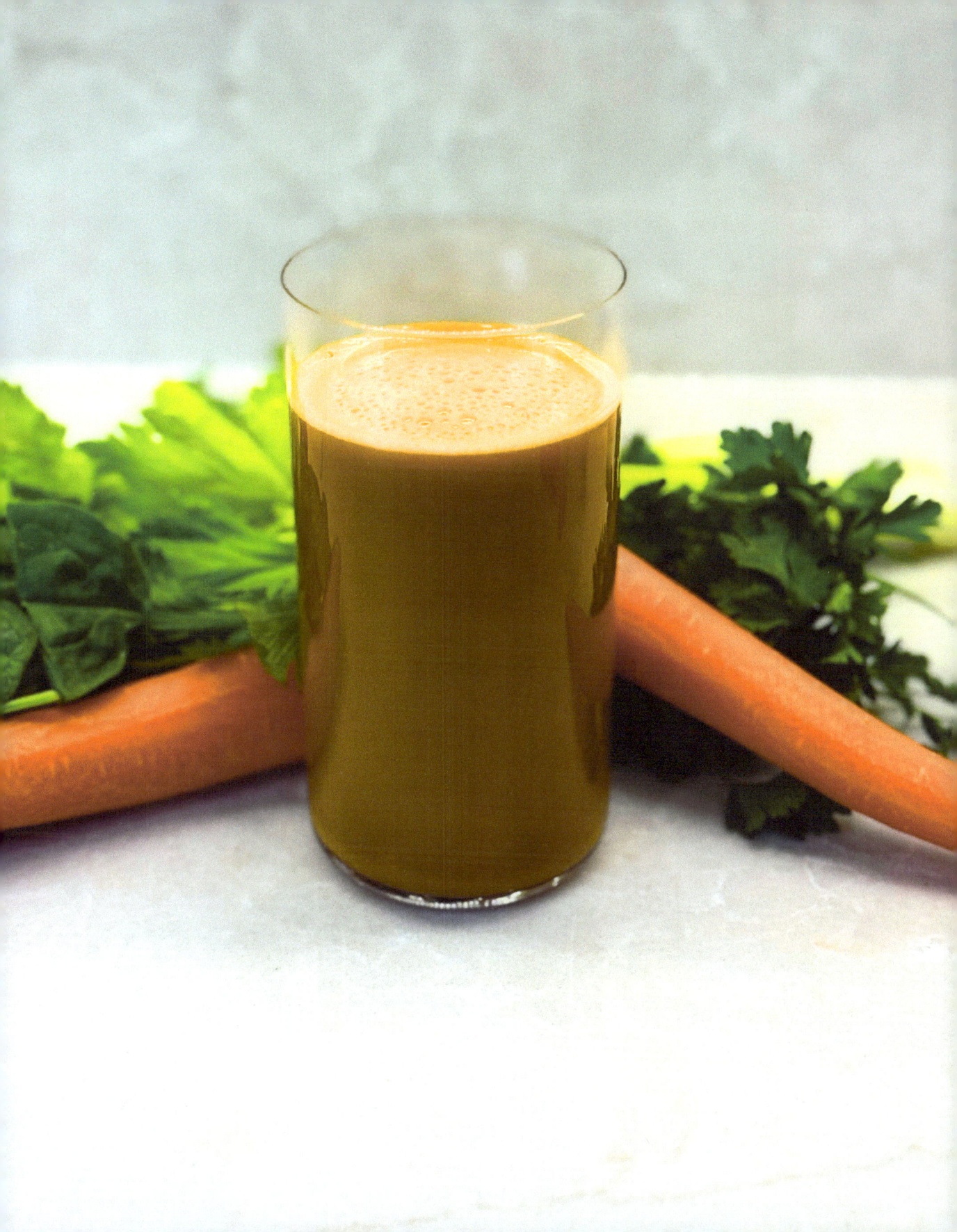

elixirs

2 ounce shots

Flu Shot:
- 1 lemon
- 4 knobs of ginger
- 2 knobs of turmeric
- black pepper

Holly's Hot Shot
- ¼ apple
- 4 knobs of ginger
- 1 lemon
- 2 knobs of turmeric

PLT
- 1 chunk of pineapple
- 1 lemon
- 2 knobs of turmeric

Chlorophyl Shot
- ¼ teaspoon of chlorella powder
- 2 ounces of filtered water

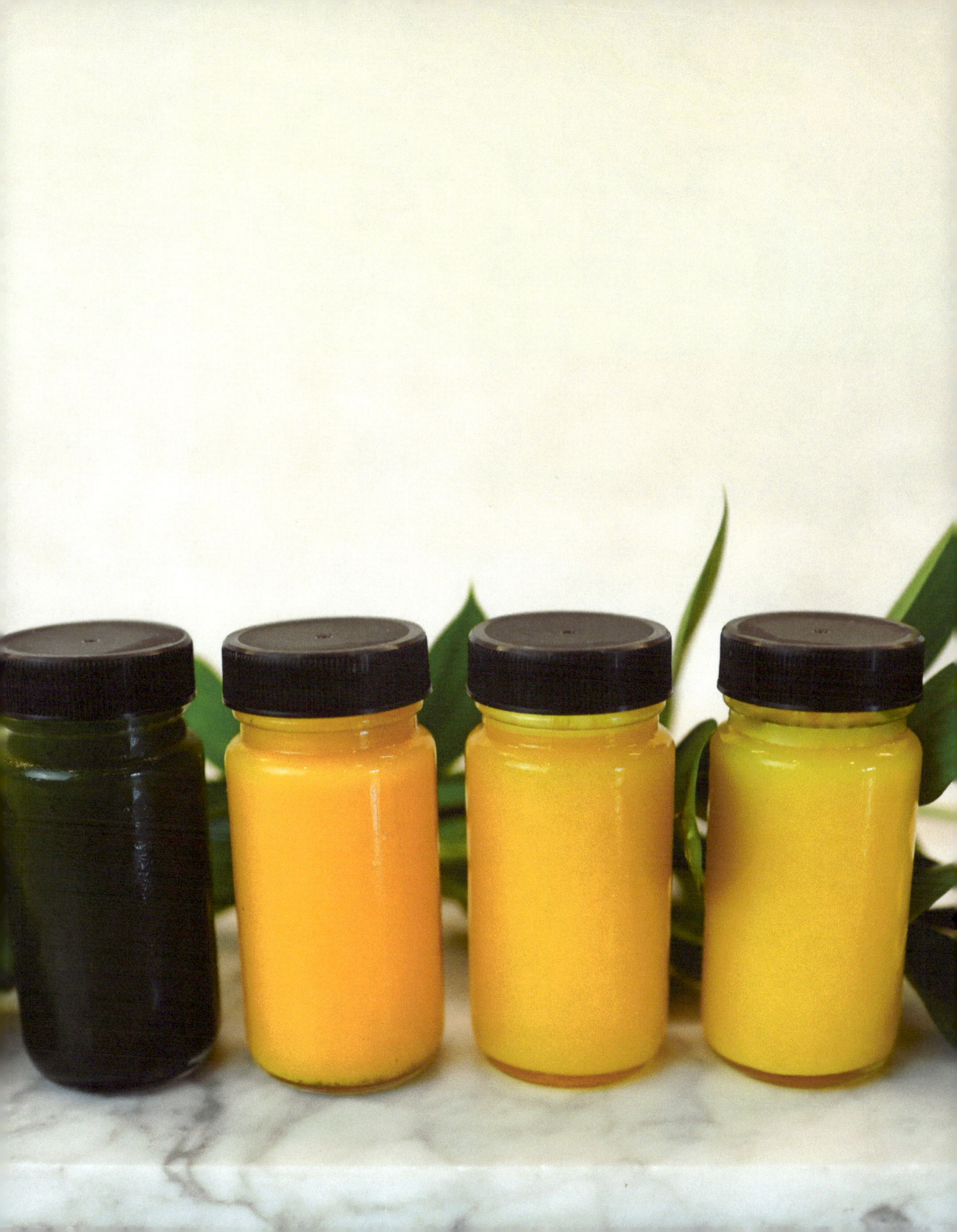

smoothies

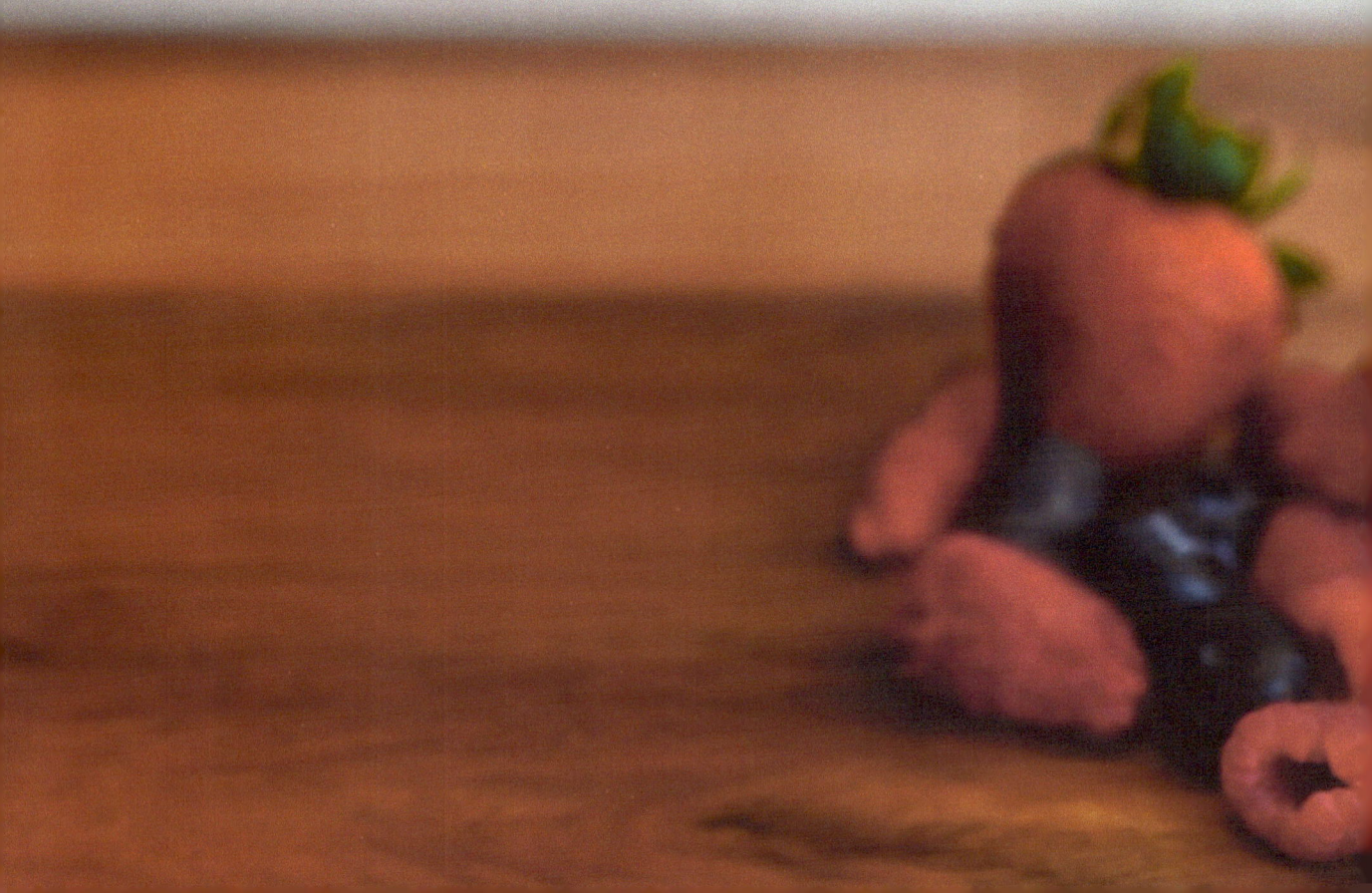

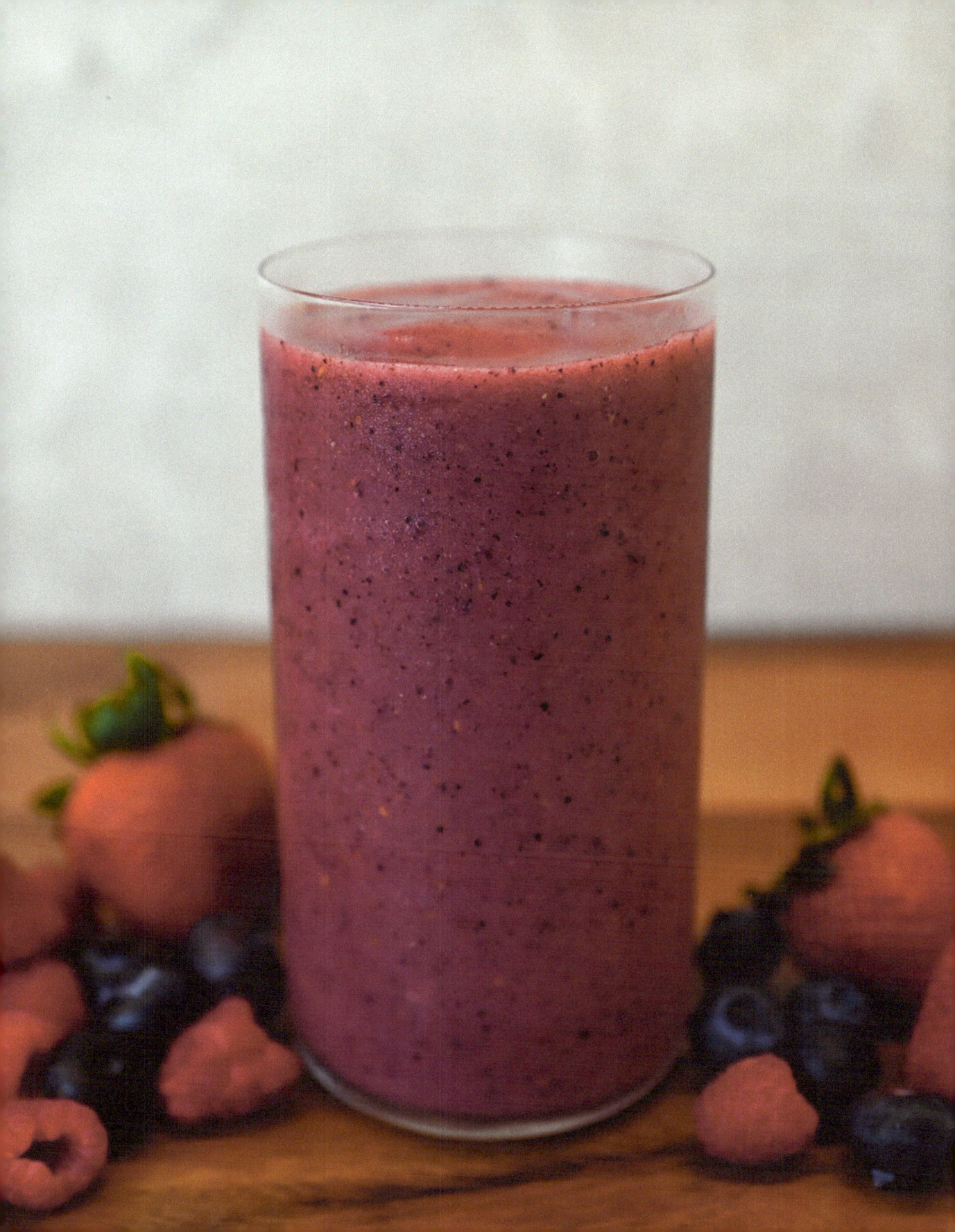

SMOOTHIE TIPS

Blender Choice:

For the best results, use a high-quality blender. Over the years, Holly has tried many, and she finds the Vitamix Vita-Prep 3 to be the most efficient. This high-power blender has a 64oz BPA-free container, making it perfect for large batches. Any Vitamix model will work well, but if you plan to make açaí or smoothie bowls, look for one with a slim base for better consistency.

Frozen Fruit:

- Always use frozen fruit instead of ice to keep your smoothie thick and cold without watering it down.

- Freeze your bananas: Peel, break them into 1-inch pieces, lay flat, and freeze. Store in a zip-lock bag, silicone storage bag, or storage containers.

Freeze Tip:

If you have leftover fresh fruit, pre-assemble your smoothie in a container or silicone bag, so it's ready to grab and blend on busy days.

Unsweetened Milks:

Use unsweetened plant-based milks to avoid added sugars. Look for milks with minimal ingredients, or you can make your own!

Add Greens

For a nutritional boost, add a handful of spinach or kale. They blend well and are nearly undetectable in taste. You can sneak greens into your family's smoothies by serving them in colored cups.

Protein Boost:

Consider adding a scoop of protein powder or a spoonful of nut butter for extra protein. If you add protein, you might want to skip sweeteners like agave, depending on the sweetness of your protein powder (Holly uses Truvanni protein, which is sweetened with monk fruit, so she doesn't need additional sweeteners).

Insider Information:

When training at the café, the items were handcrafted as they were ordered. All employees learned how to make all the recipes without measuring. They did use a reference board for ingredients, but everyone added the items to the blender or juicer without measuring. This allowed us to make the recipes efficiently, ensuring for the fastest ticket time possible. As you master the art of handcrafting the recipes yourself, you should be able to "graduate" from measuring, which will save you time.

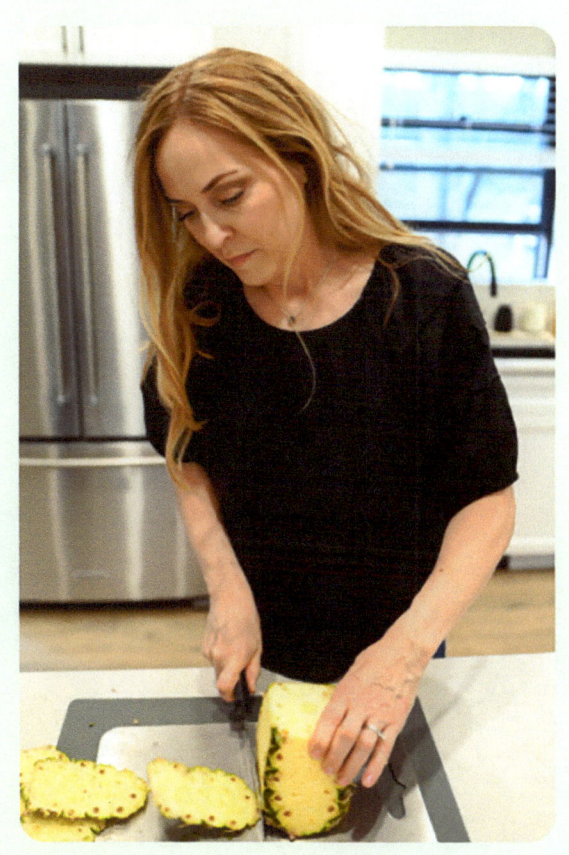

BLENDING PROCESS

Blending Process:

Add all your ingredients to the blender, secure the lid, and start on a low speed, gradually increasing to high. Blend until smooth and creamy.

- If your smoothie is too thick, add a bit more liquid.

- If it's too thin, add more frozen fruit. (This can happen if your fruit isn't fully frozen or if the measurements were off.)

If you have air pockets in the bottom of the blender, you aren't filling it all up and it'll be more liquidy. So be sure that the frozen fruit is spread evenly in the blender.

Holly realizes nut milk isn't for everyone. If you use regular milk, keep in mind it tends to blend up with a creamy, frothy finish. Use less real milk to start, as you many need less due to the different consistency.

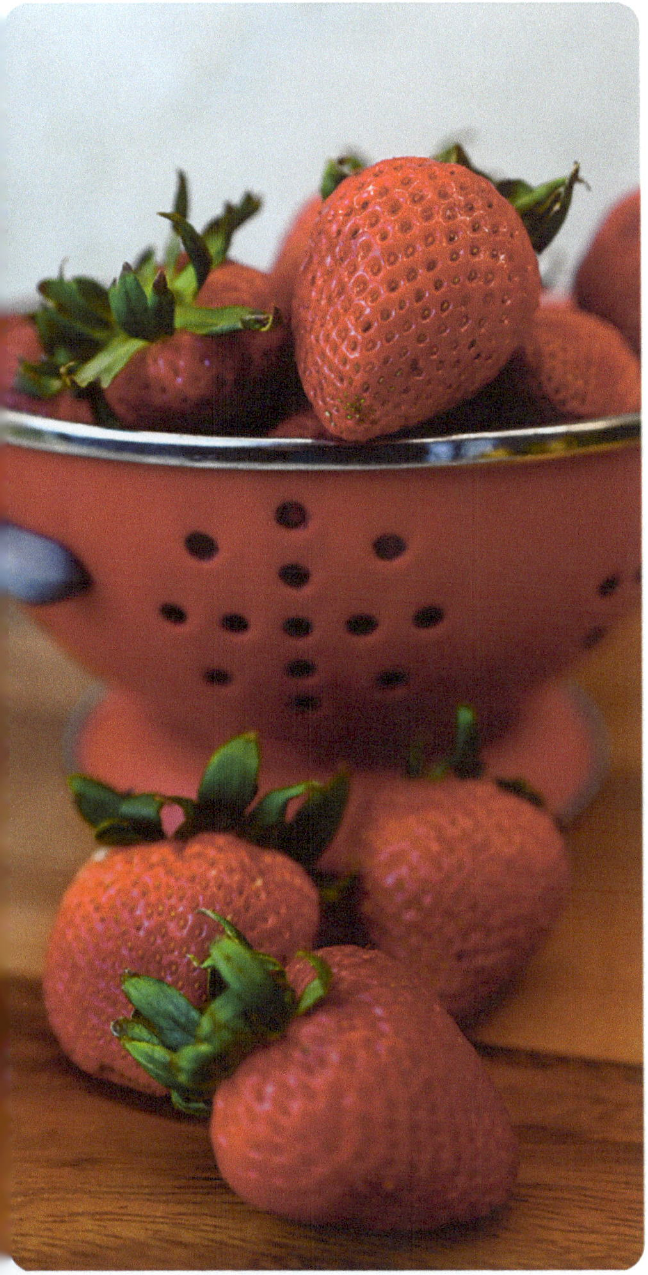

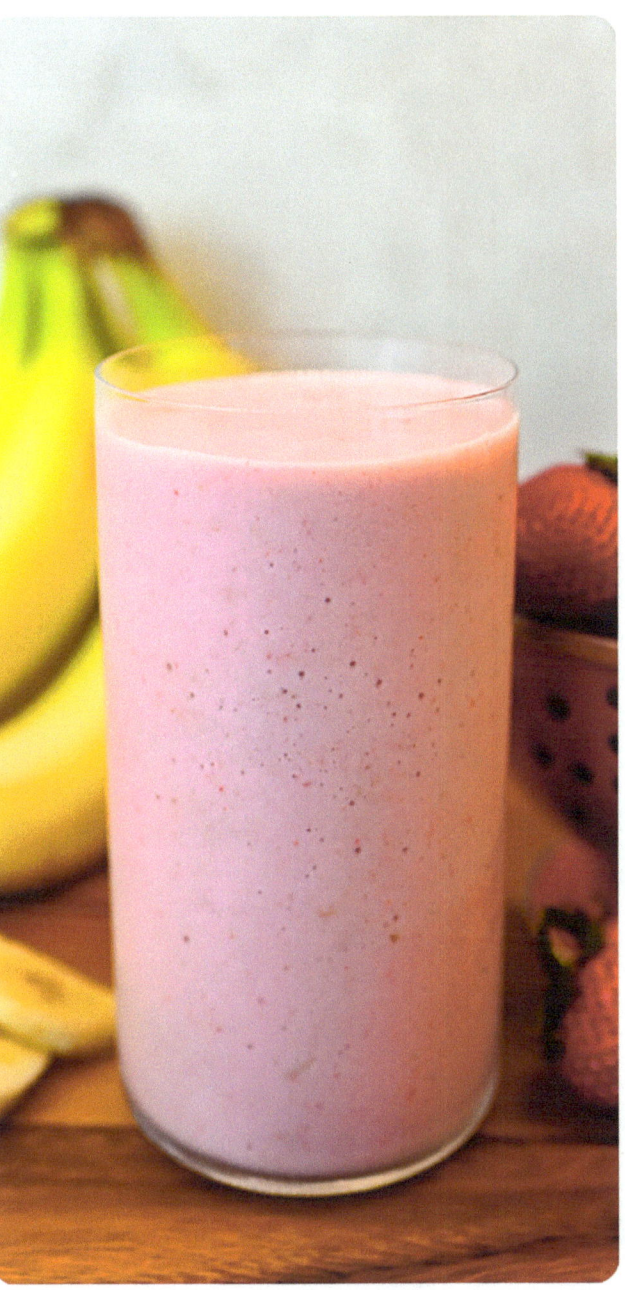

almondbuttercrunch

Ingredients

- 1 cup oat milk
- 1.5 cups frozen banana
- 1 tablespoon almond butter
- 2 tablespoons cacao nibs
- 1 teaspoon maca

Instructions

1. Add all the ingredients to a blender.
2. Blend until smooth and creamy.
3. Pour into a glass and enjoy immediately!

This smoothie was done as a special and we always had to brace ourselves and make sure we were stocked up on almond butter and oat milk. This smoothie was the top selling special smoothie.

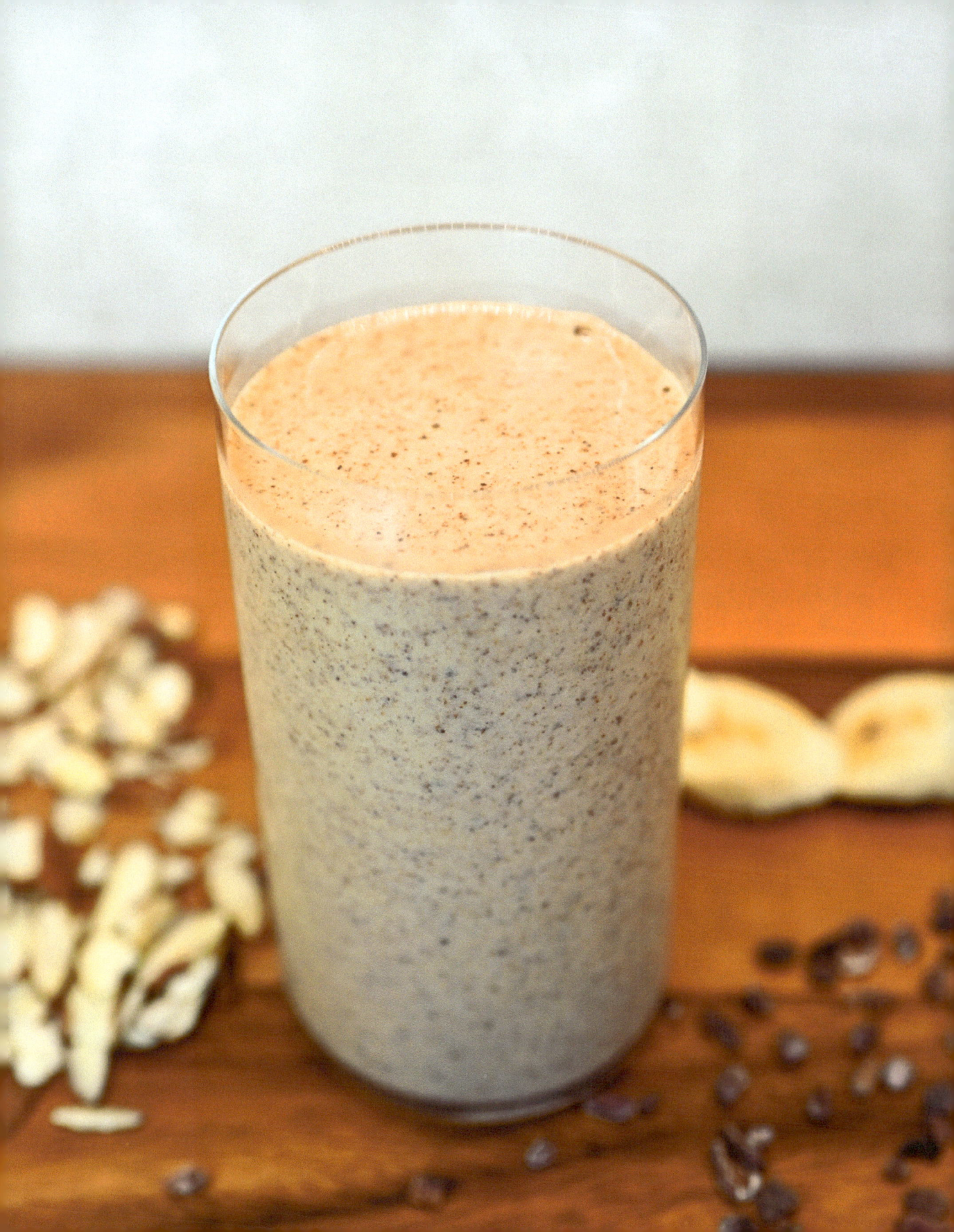

berry**bunch**

smoothie

Ingredients

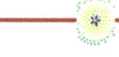

- 1 cup coconut water
- ⅓ cup frozen blueberries
- ⅓ cup frozen strawberries
- ⅓ cup frozen raspberries
- 1 teaspoon maca

Instructions

1. Add all the ingredients to a blender.
2. Blend until smooth and creamy.
3. Pour into a glass and enjoy immediately!

TIPS

 Pairs well with hemp or vanilla protein

 Spinach and Kale can be hidden in this one easily.

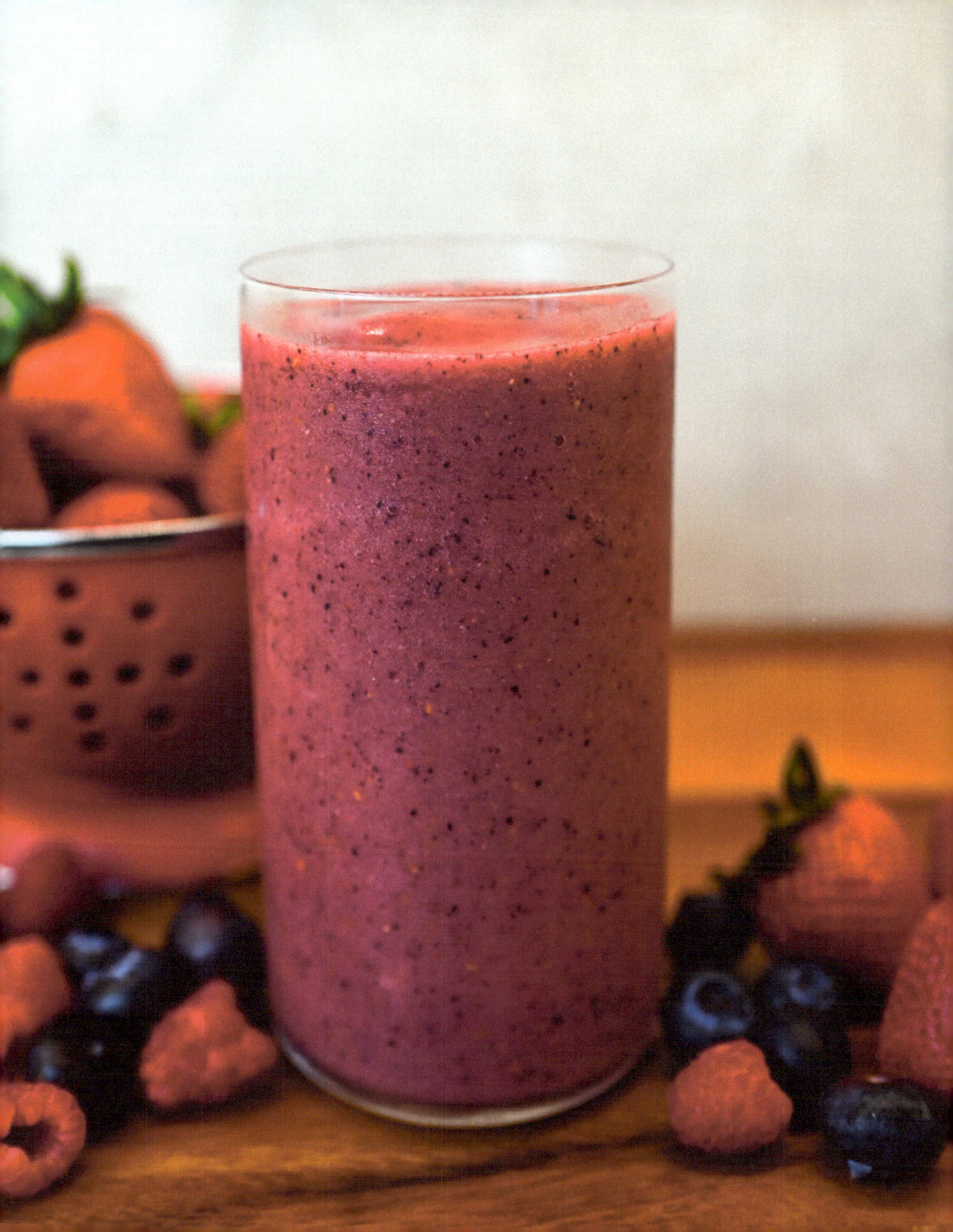

blueberrybananabliss

This smoothie was never on the menu, but Holly created it for a famous someone who often stopped by.

Ingredients

- 1 cup almond milk
- ½ cup frozen blueberries
- ½ cup frozen banana
- 1 tablespoon almond butter
- 2 handfuls spinach
- 1 serving of vanilla protein

Instructions

1. Add all the ingredients to a blender.
2. Blend until smooth and creamy.
3. Pour into a glass and enjoy immediately!

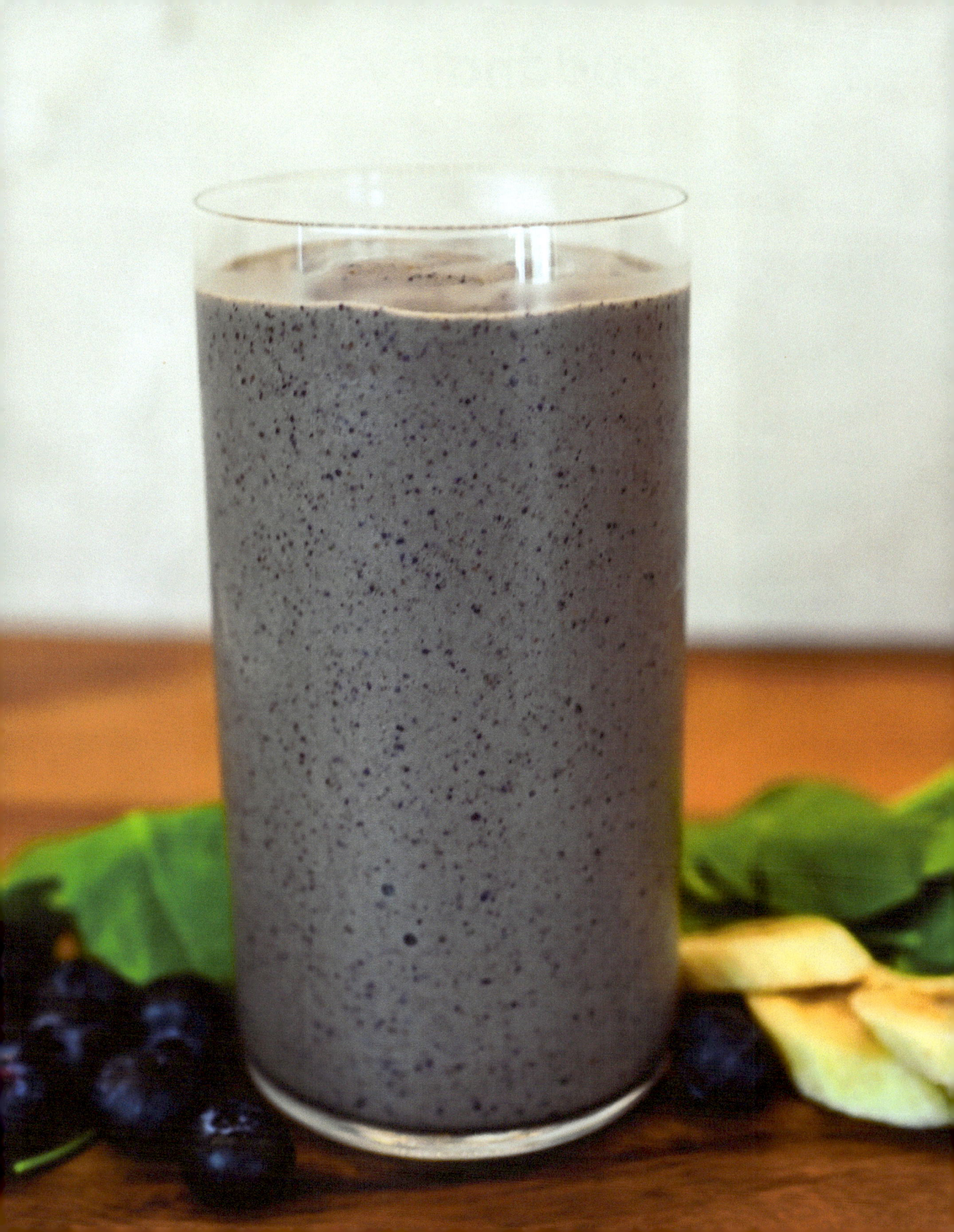

buddhalove

smoothie

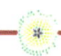

We can't describe it; other than it tastes like LOVE.

Ingredients

- 1 cup almond milk
- ¾ cup frozen banana
- ¼ cup coconut meat
- 2 tablespoons goji berries
- 1 tablespoon almond butter
- 1 teaspoon vanilla extract
- 1 teaspoon agave

Instructions

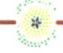

1. Add all the ingredients to a blender.
2. Blend until smooth and creamy.
3. Pour into a glass and enjoy immediately!

TIPS

 Add vanilla protein

 If you don't want banana, this works well with blueberries.

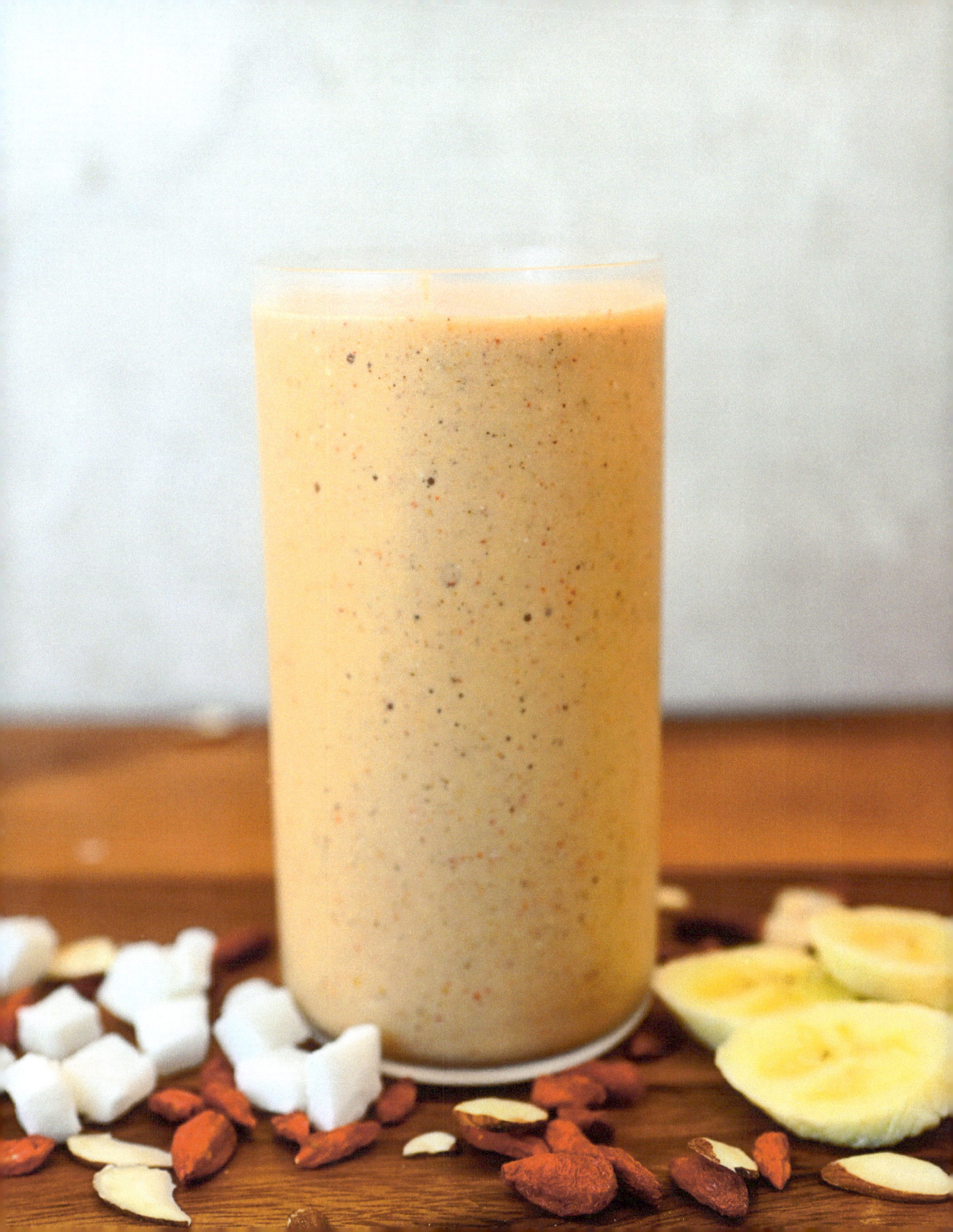

chocolatepowersmoothie

Ingredients

- 1 cup of almond milk
- 1.5 cups frozen banana
- 1 scoop of chocolate protein
- 1 teaspoon of cacao powder
- 1 teaspoon of almond butter

Instructions

1. Add all the ingredients to a blender.
2. Blend until smooth and creamy.
3. Pour into a glass and enjoy immediately!

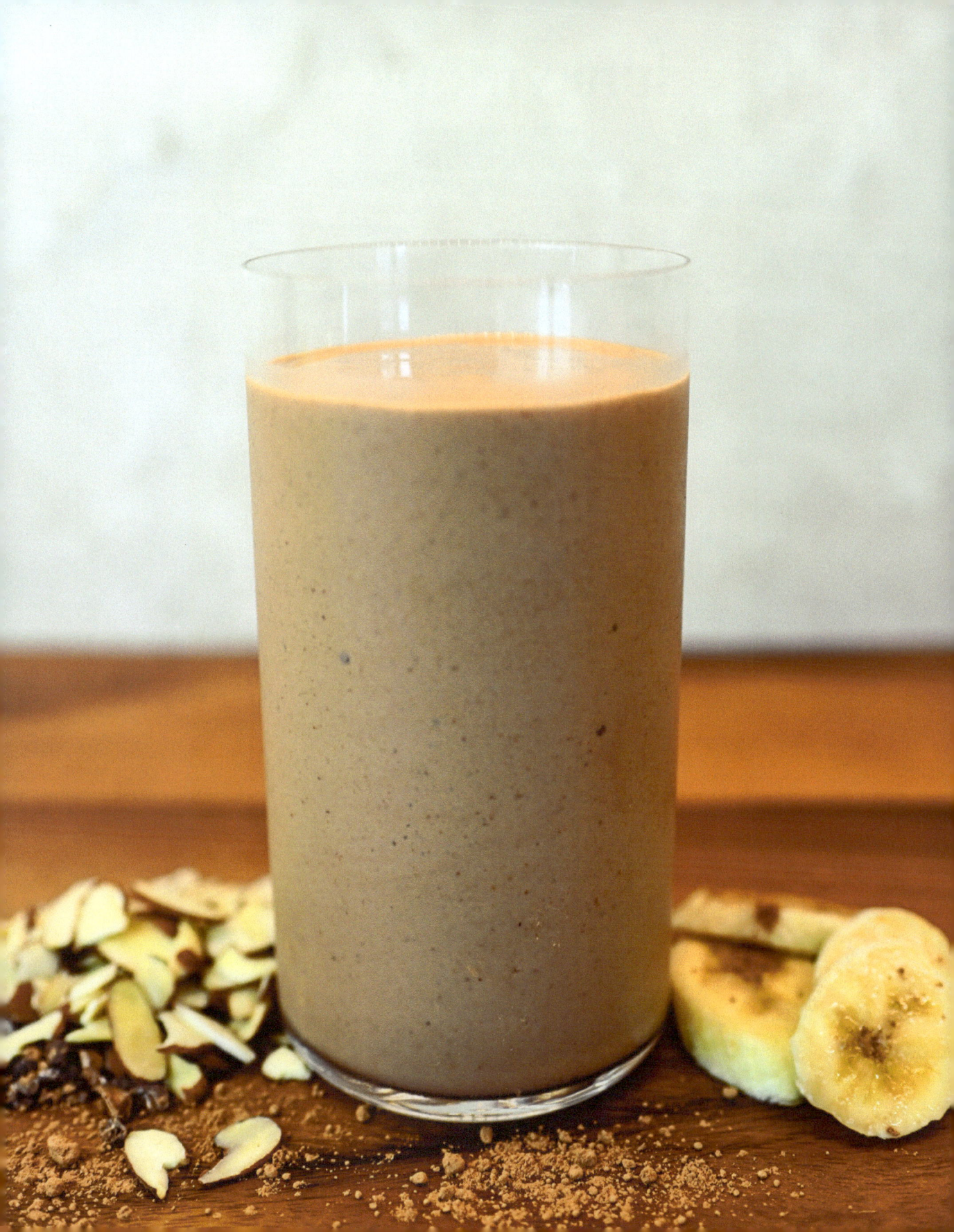

funkymonkey

Ingredients

- 1 cup almond milk
- ¾ cup frozen banana
- 1 tablespoon peanut butter
- 1 serving size of chocolate protein powder

Originally, this had a choice of vanilla or chocolate protein. We switched it to just chocolate to speed up the ordering process. We would sub vanilla for anyone who asked.

Instructions

1. Add all the ingredients to a blender.
2. Blend until smooth and creamy.
3. Pour into a glass and enjoy immediately!

TIP

 The funkymoney smoothie is excellent with almond butter!

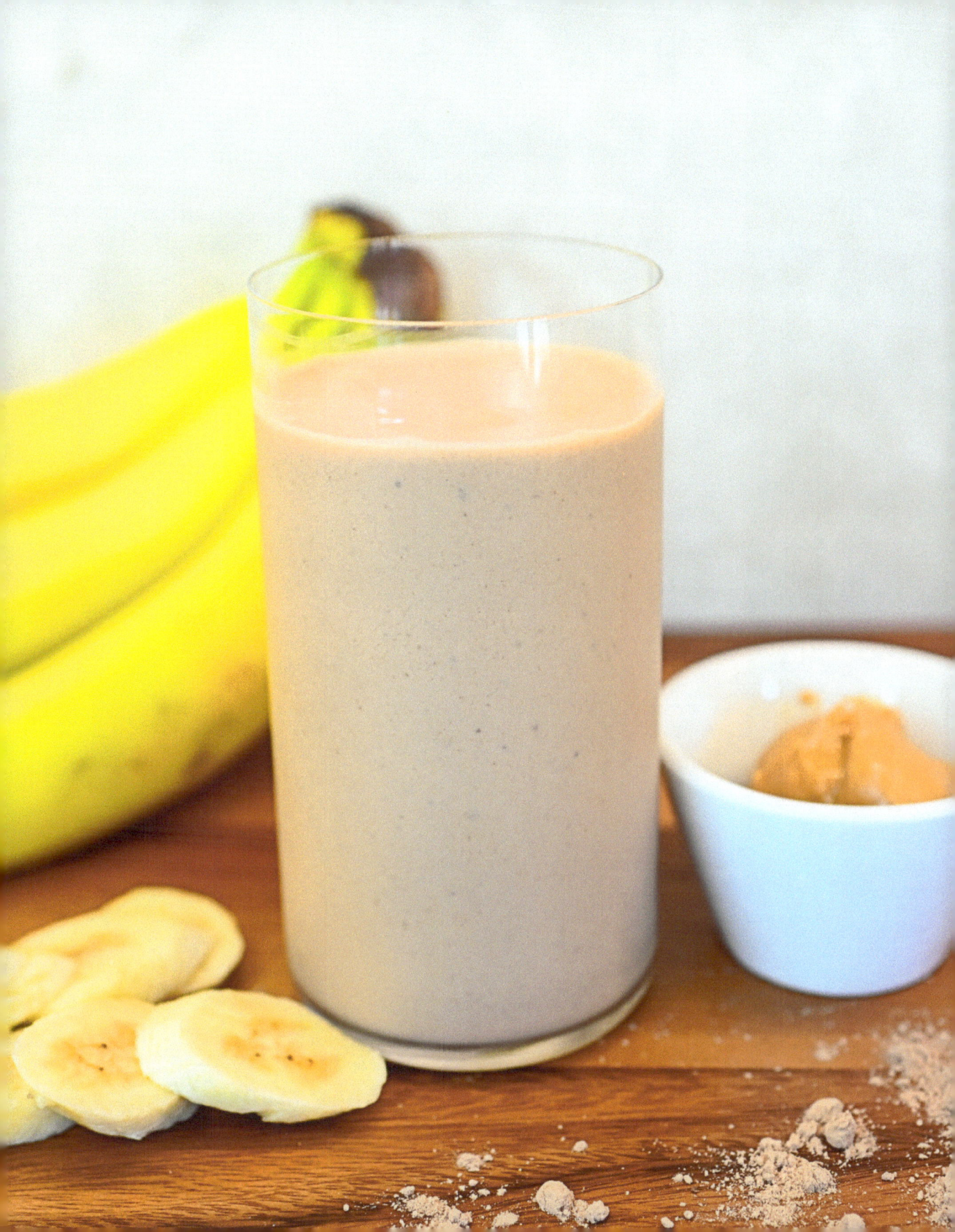

littleapple

smoothie

Ingredients

- 1 cup almond milk
- ½ cup frozen apple
- ½ cup frozen banana
- 1 large kale leaf
- 2 ounces goji berries
- 1 tablespoon honey

Instructions

1. Add all the ingredients to a blender.
2. Blend until smooth and creamy.
3. Pour into a glass and enjoy immediately!

TIPS

 Add vanilla protein

 Always put your kale on top of your frozen fruit.

 Great for breakfast or a mid-morning snack

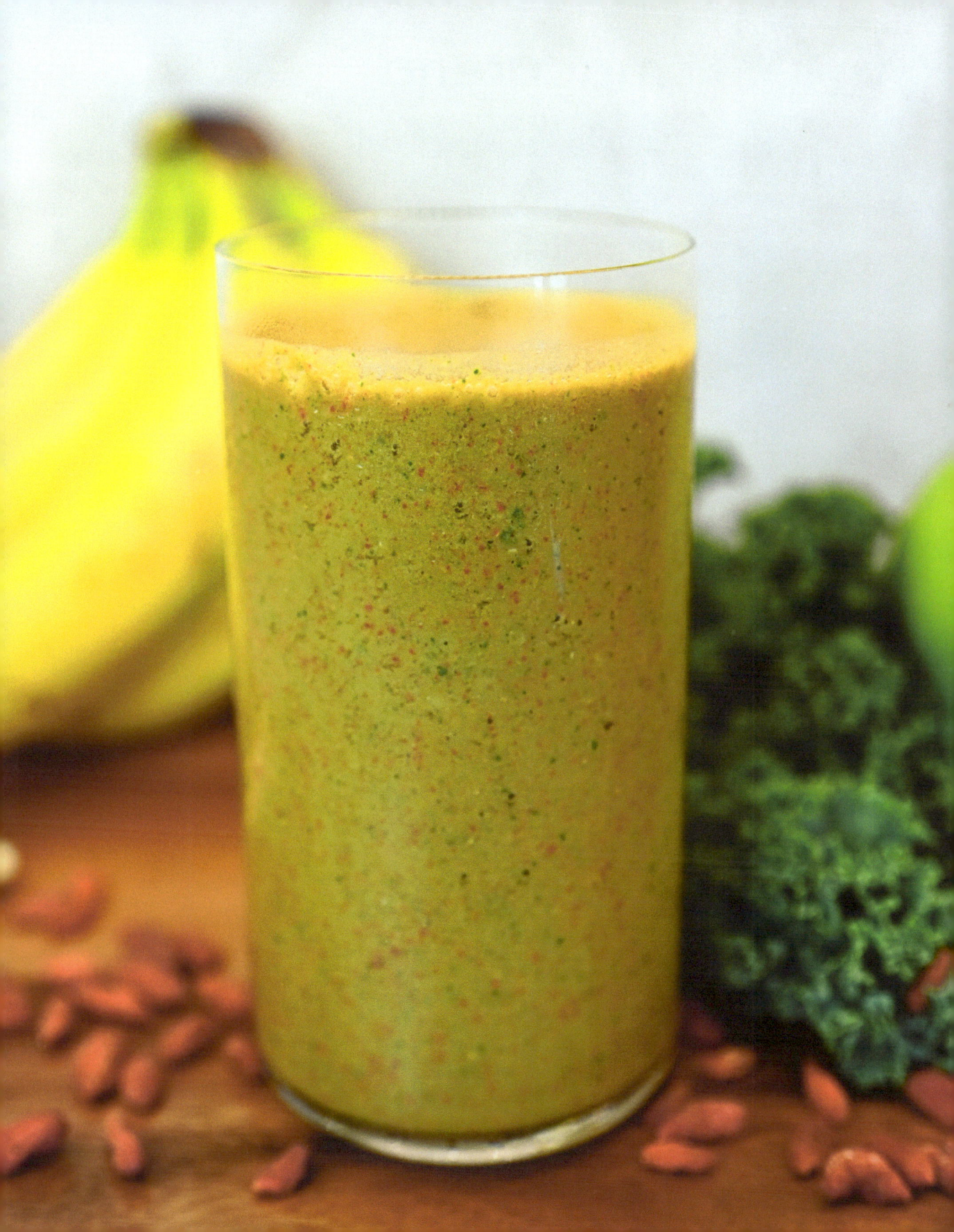

macarena

smoothie

Every now an then someone would order this smoothie by signing the song.

Ingredients

- 1 cup oat milk
- ¾ cup frozen banana
- 1 tablespoon almond butter
- ¼ cup coconut meat (raw)
- 1 teaspoon cacao
- 1 teaspoon maca
- 2 dates

Instructions

1. Add all the ingredients to a blender.
2. Blend until smooth and creamy.
3. Pour into a glass and enjoy immediately!

TIP

 Pairs well with chocolate or vanilla protein

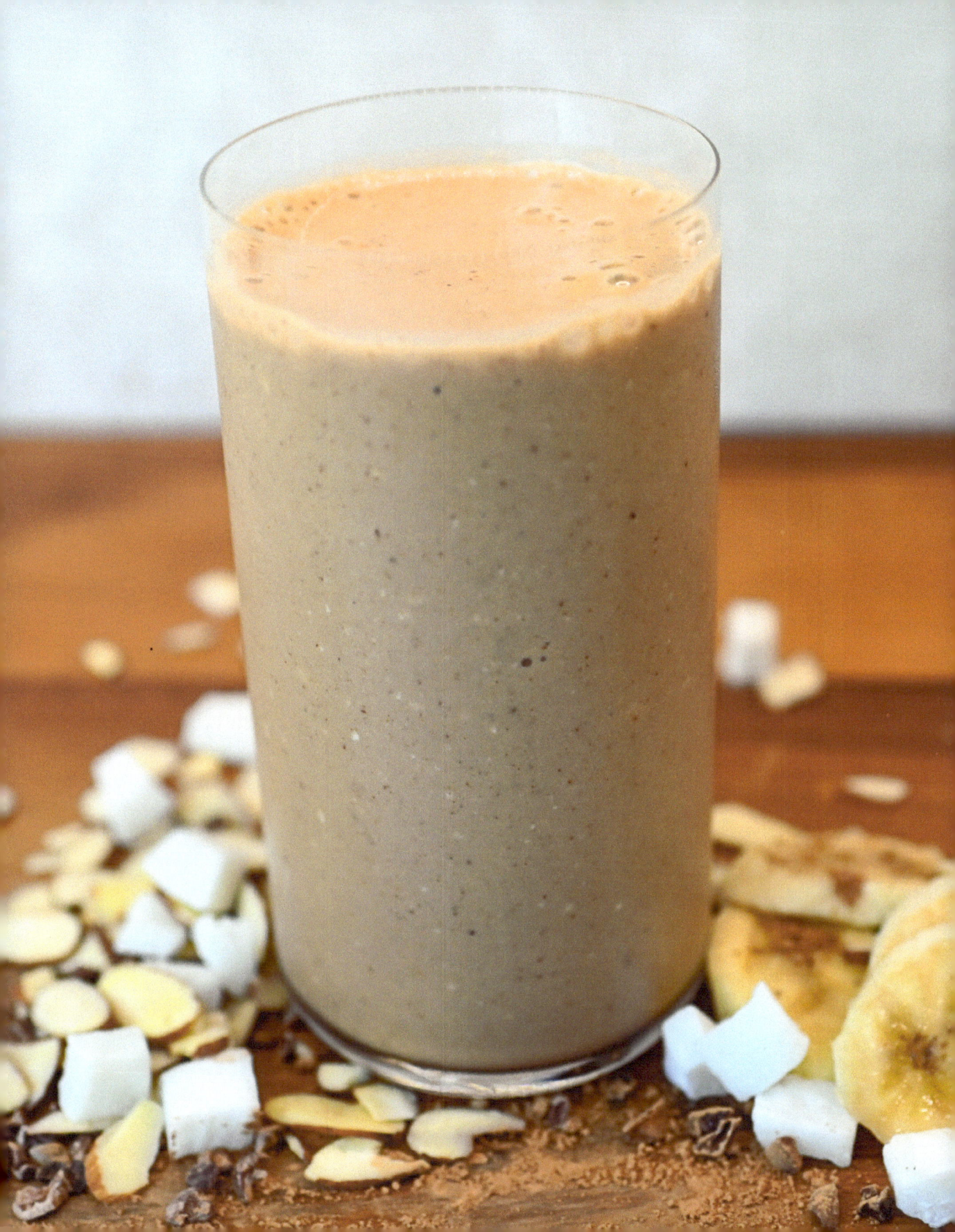

marytylermoringa

smoothie

marytylermoringa smoothie is refreshing and on the lighter side. Great for hot days.

Ingredients

- 1 cup coconut water
- ⅓ cup frozen mango
- ⅓ cup frozen pineapple
- ⅓ cup frozen strawberries
- 1 teaspoon moringa

Instructions

1. Add all the ingredients to a blender.
2. Blend until smooth and creamy.
3. Pour into a glass and enjoy immediately!

TIP

 You can't taste the morninga. It's really good for you, so why not have it.

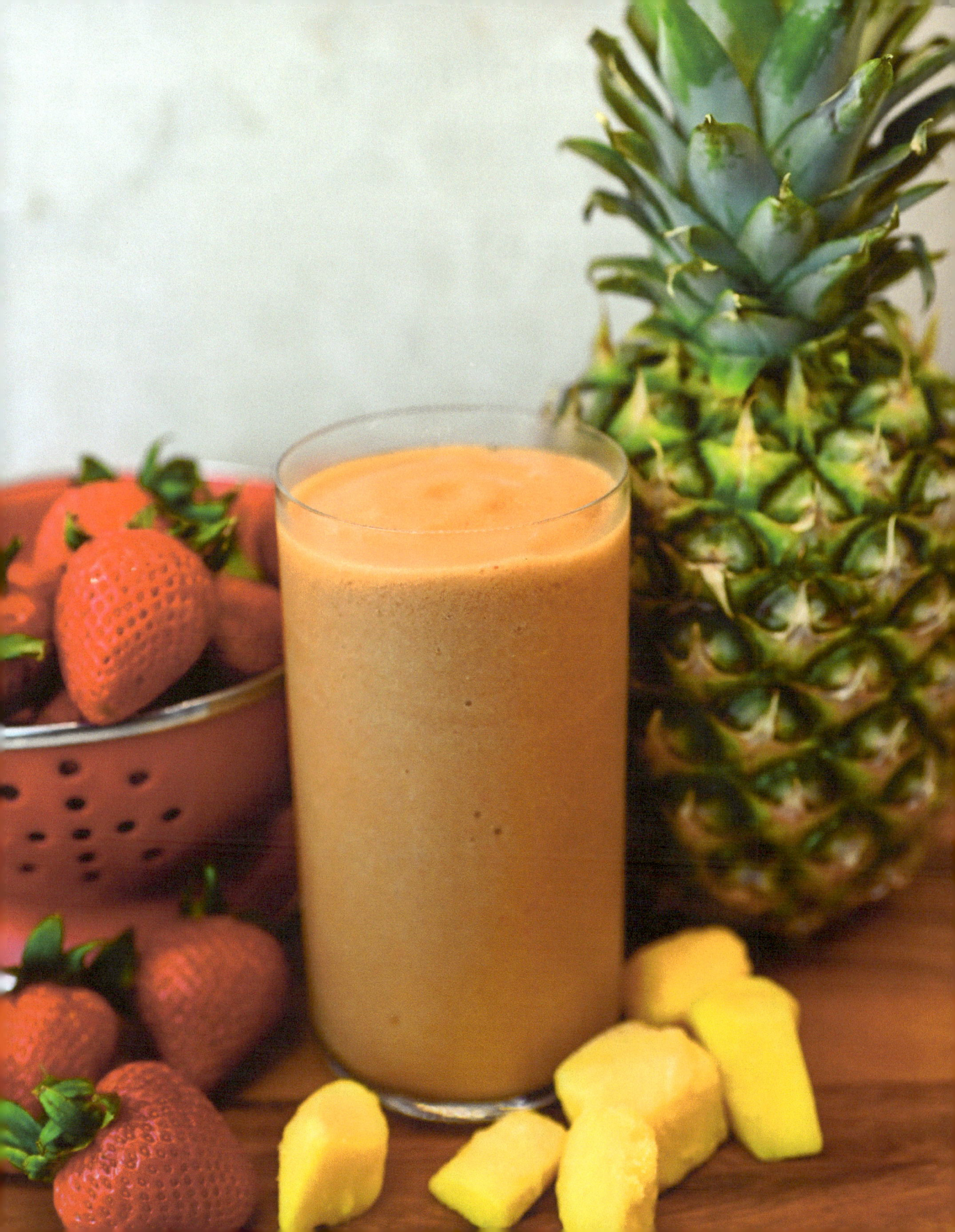

midnightexpress

smoothie

Freeze any leftover coffee in ice cube trays to use in this recipe.

Ingredients

- ¼ cup oat milk
- ¾ cup iced coffee
- ¾ cup frozen banana
- 2 ounces cashews
- 2 dates
- 1 teaspoon vanilla

Instructions

1. Add all the ingredients to a blender.
2. Blend until smooth and creamy.
3. Pour into a glass and enjoy immediately!

TIPS

 If you have extra coffee, keep it in the fridge to use in your midnight express.

 Pairs well with chocolate protein

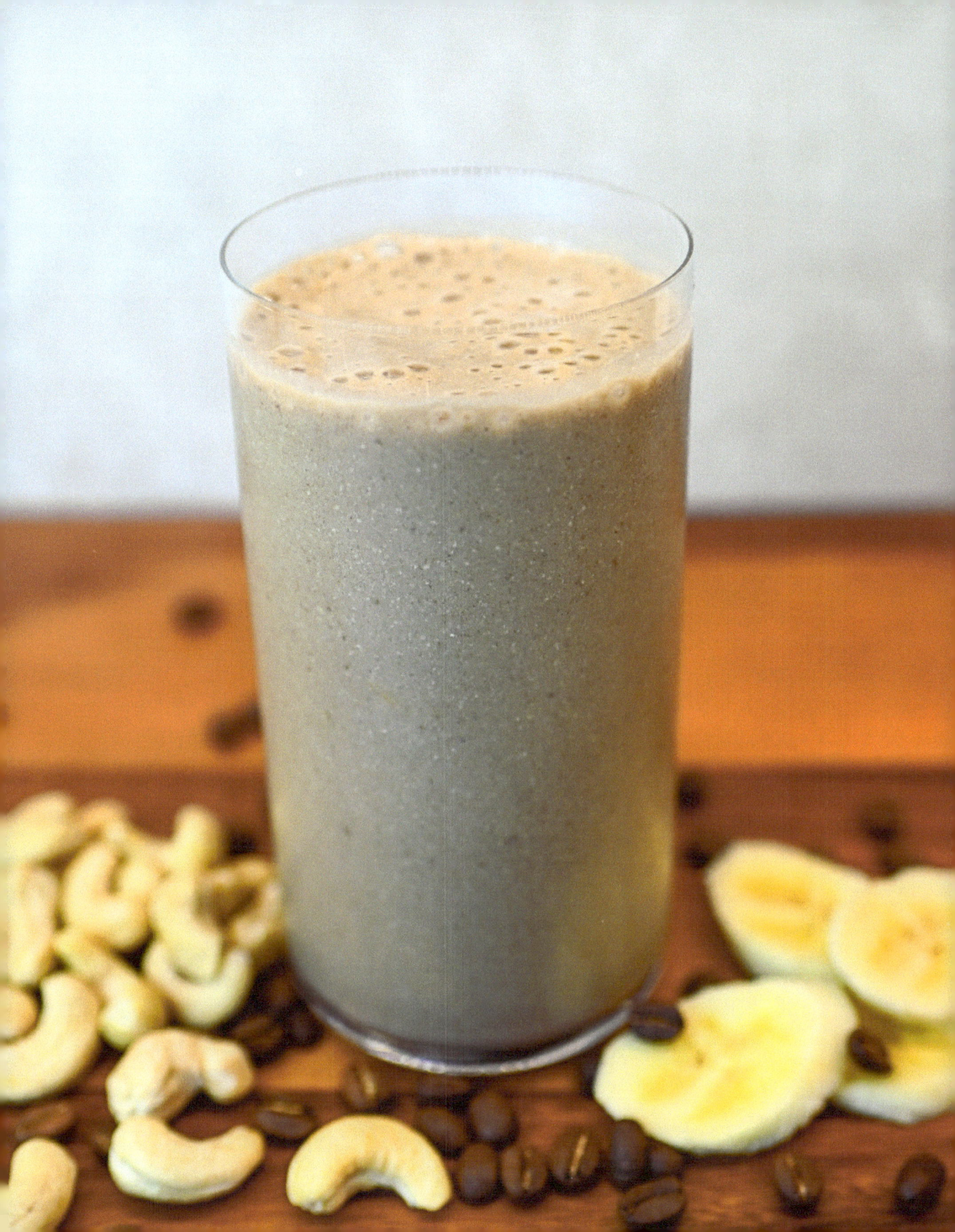

peacepunch

Ingredients

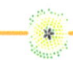

- 1 cup oat milk
- ½ cup frozen pineapple
- ½ cup frozen banana
- 3 mint stems
- 1 knob ginger

Instructions

1. Add all the ingredients to a blender.
2. Blend until smooth and creamy.
3. Pour into a glass and enjoy immediately!

TIP

✽ Add vanilla protein

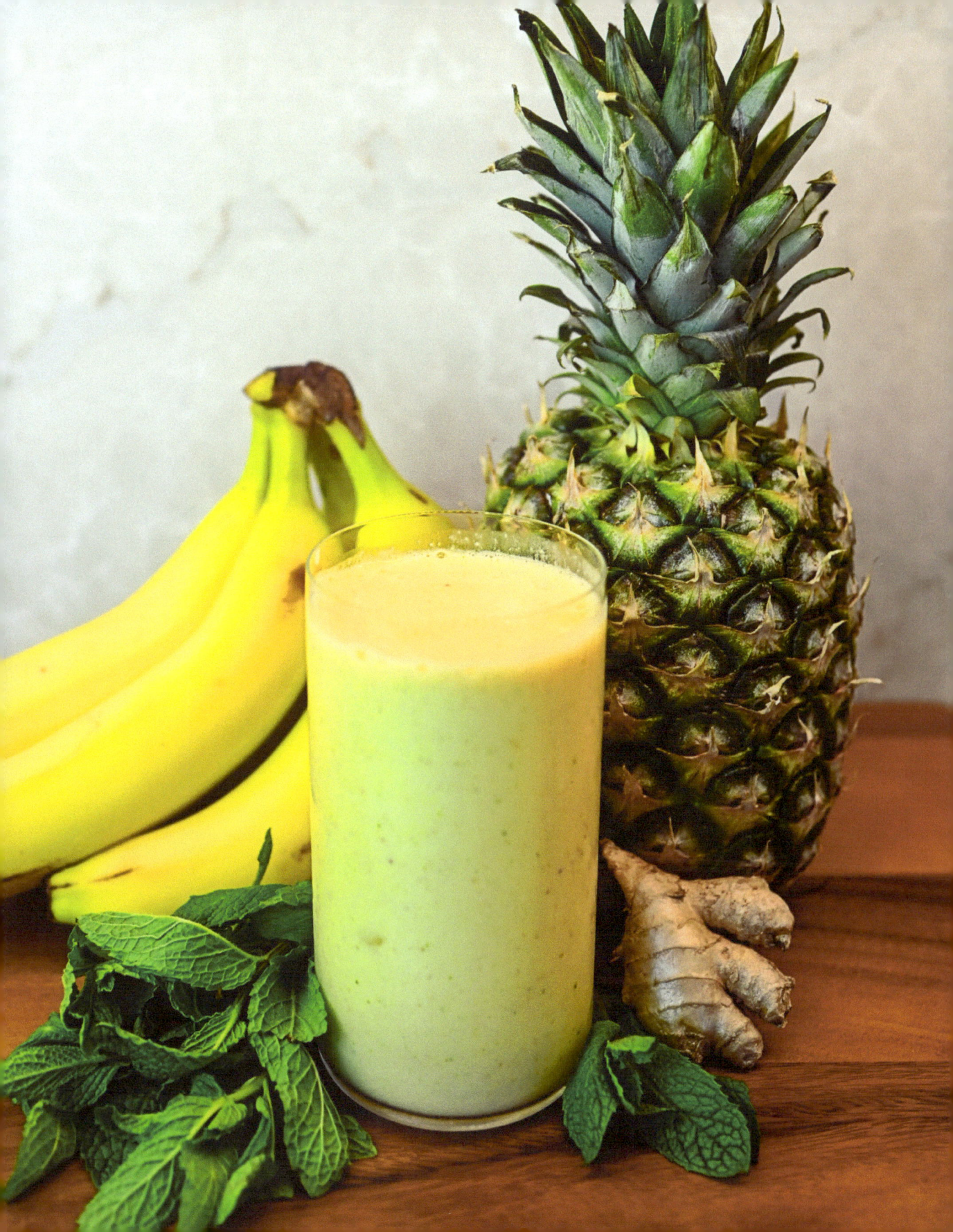

peanutbuttercrunch

smoothie

Ingredients

- 1 cup almond milk
- 1.5 cups banana
- 1 tablespoon peanut butter
- 2 tablespoons of raw peanuts

Instructions

1. Add all the ingredients to a blender.
2. Blend until smooth and creamy.
3. Pour into a glass and enjoy immediately!

TIP

 Pairs well with chocolate protein

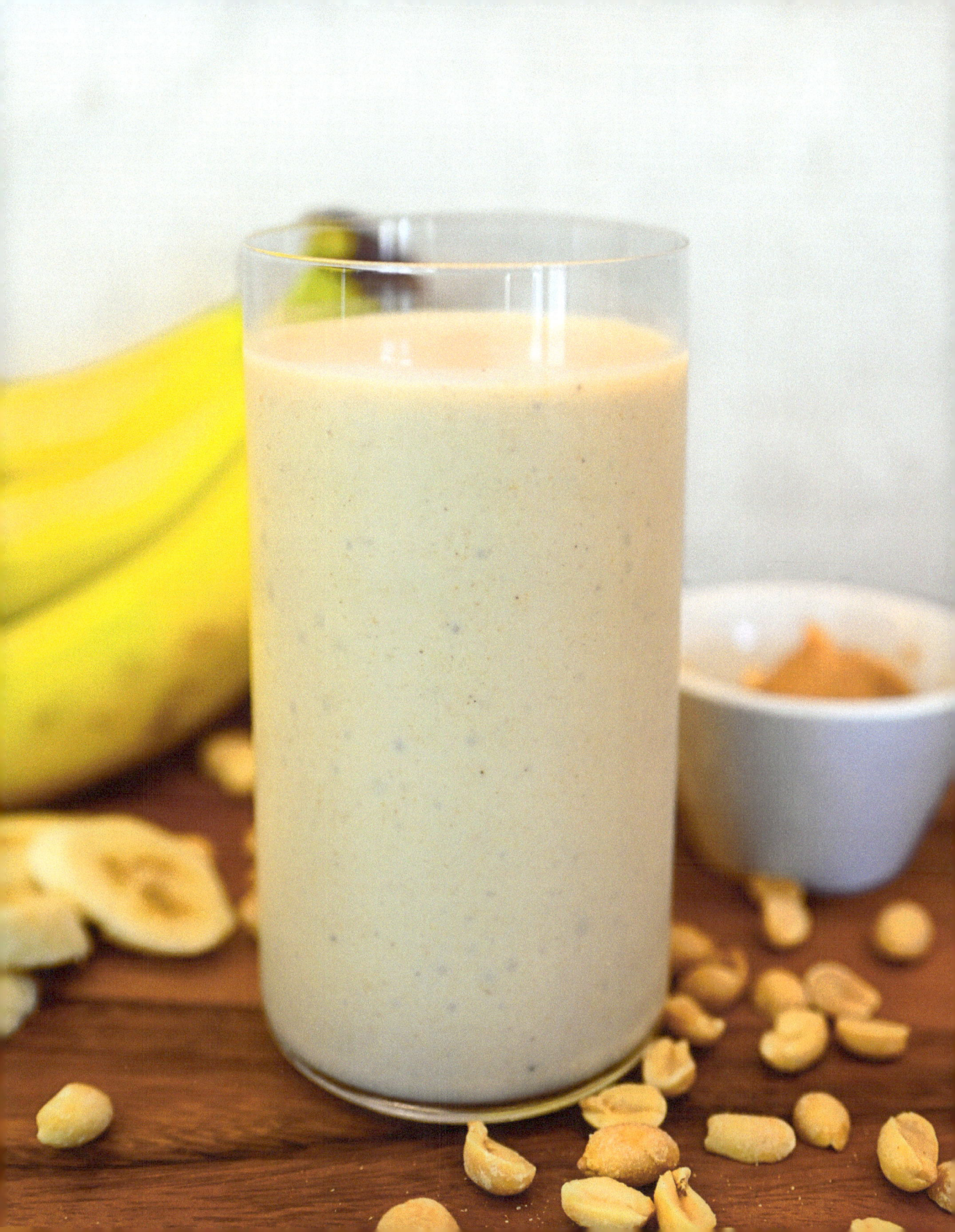

pineapple paradise
smoothie

We had a staff member love this smoothie so much we gave her a blender when she went off to college so she could continue to make it.

Ingredients

- ½ cup pineapple juice
- ½ cup coconut milk
- ½ cup frozen pineapple
- ½ cup frozen mango
- 1 teaspoon agave

Instructions

1. Add all the ingredients to a blender.
2. Blend until smooth and creamy.
3. Pour into a glass and enjoy immediately!

TIPS

 Pairs well with vanilla protein

 If you don't have pineapple juice, feel free to use coconut milk instead. You can also stick with just pineapple juice—just be sure to skip the agave to keep it from getting too sweet.

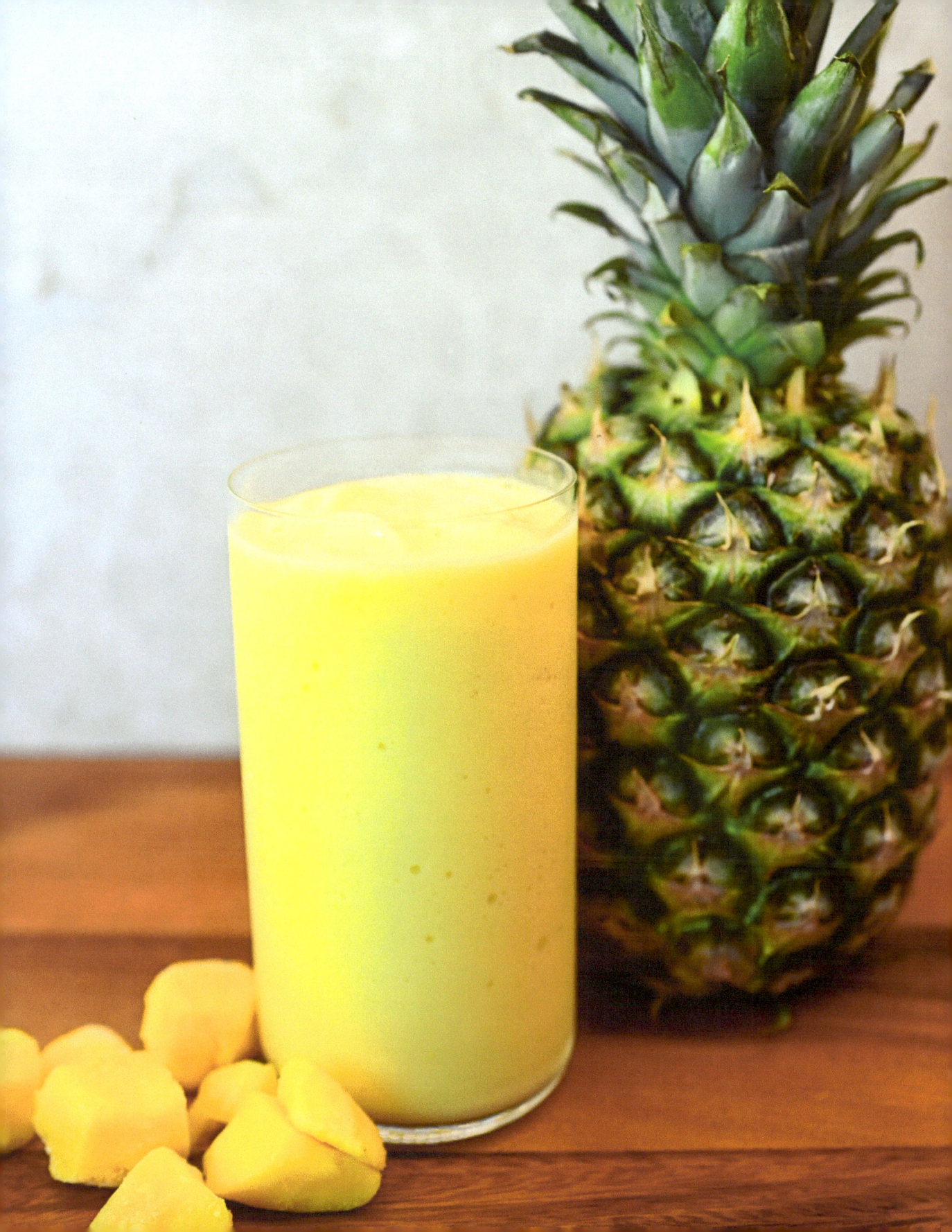

scrumptiousstrawberry

smoothie

Ingredients

- 1 cup almond milk
- ½ cup frozen strawberry
- ½ cup frozen banana
- 1 teaspoon cinnamon
- 1 teaspoon vanilla extract
- 1 teaspoon agave

Holly created this smoothie for her son years before she had the café. It was one of the top 3 selling smoothies every year.

Instructions

1. Add all the ingredients to a blender.
2. Blend until smooth and creamy.
3. Pour into a glass and enjoy immediately!

TIPS

 Add vanilla protein

 If you don't want banana, just add all strawberries instead

 Have a fussy eater at home? Add a handful or two of spinach and serve in a colored cup. They won't be able to tell it is in there.

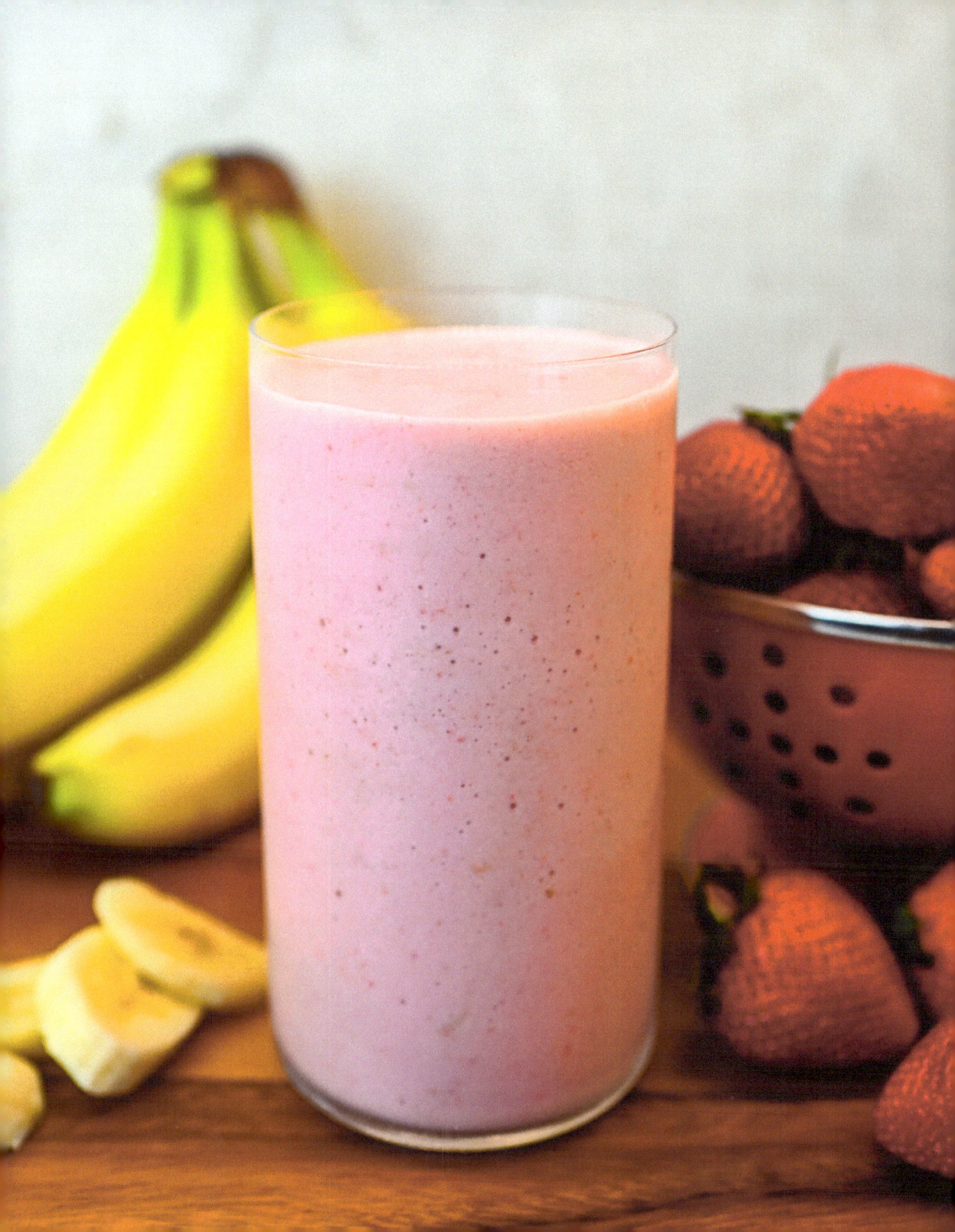

thedutchess

smoothie

This smoothie is a go to for Holly's family.

Ingredients

- ½ cup coconut water
- ½ cup frozen pineapple
- 1 orange (peeled)
- 2 handfuls spinach
- ¼ cup frozen banana

Instructions

1. Add all the ingredients to a blender.
2. Blend until smooth and creamy.
3. Pour into a glass and enjoy immediately!

TIP

 Pairs well with vanilla protein. Also, if you have a fresh lime toss one in it tastes amazing.

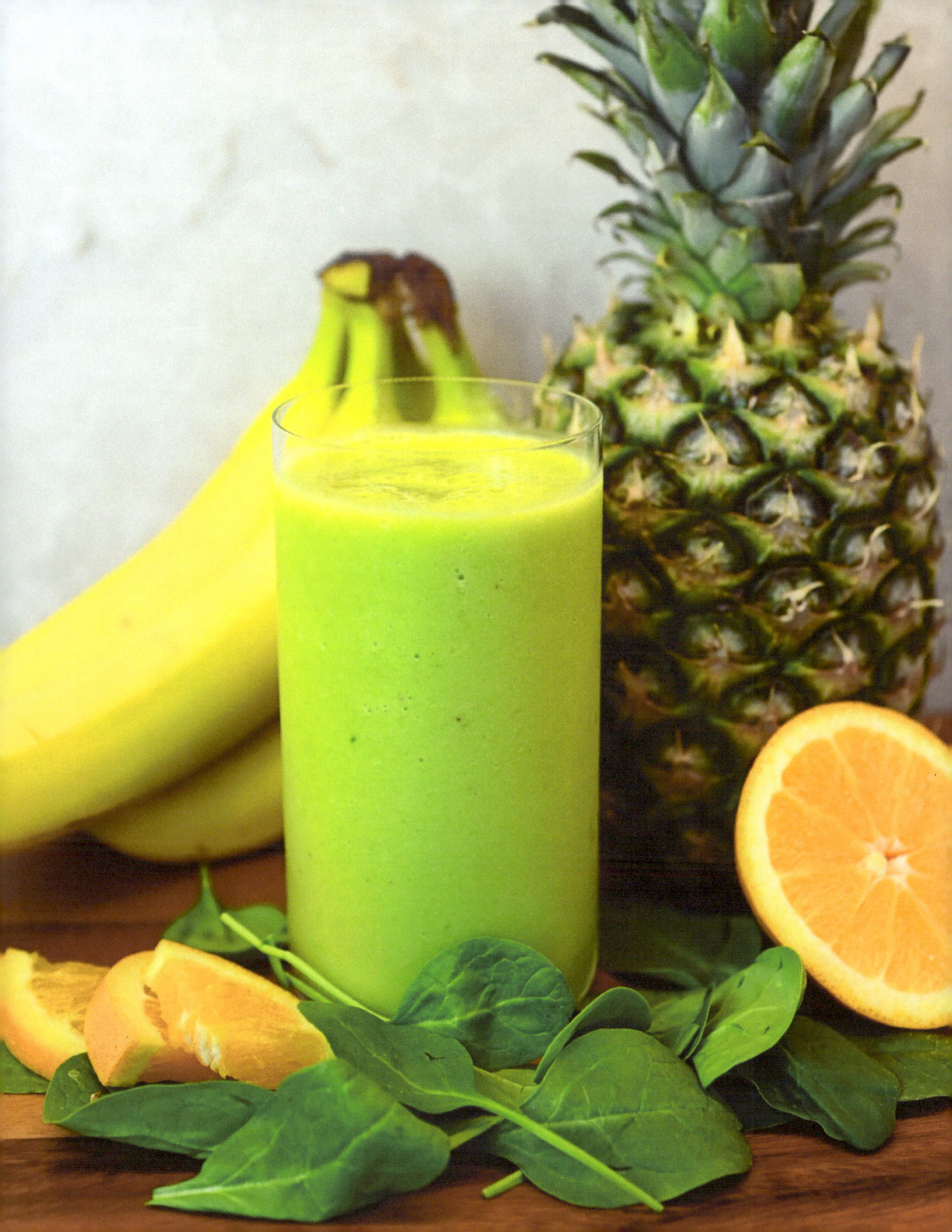

tropical**blast**

smoothie

Ingredients

- 1 cup coconut water
- ¼ cup frozen pineapple
- ¼ cup frozen blueberries
- ¼ cup frozen mango
- 1 knob ginger

Holly made this smoothie at home for years prior to owning the café. She always adds spinach.

Instructions

1. Add all the ingredients to a blender.
2. Blend until smooth and creamy.
3. Pour into a glass and enjoy immediately!

TIP

 Pairs well with spinach or kale. This smoothie hides the flavor of both well.

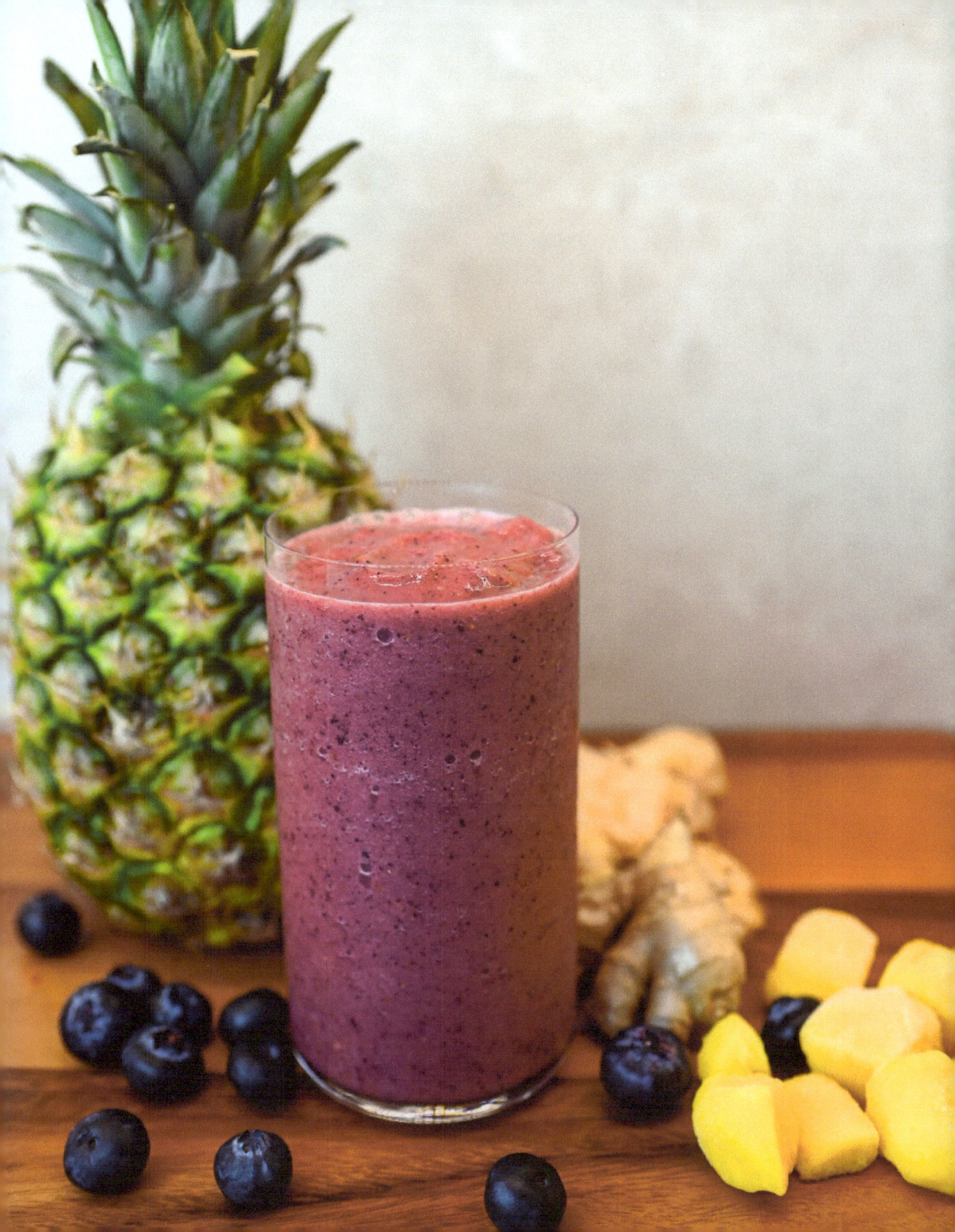

tropicalsunrise

smoothie

This smoothie was never on the menu, but to this day, it is still on Holly's morning rotation of favorite smoothies.

Ingredients

- 1 cup almond milk
- ½ cup frozen pineapple
- ½ cup frozen mango
- 1 knob ginger
- 1 serving of vanilla protein

Instructions

1. Add all the ingredients to a blender.
2. Blend until smooth and creamy.
3. Pour into a glass and enjoy immediately!

TIP

Pairs well with fresh mint

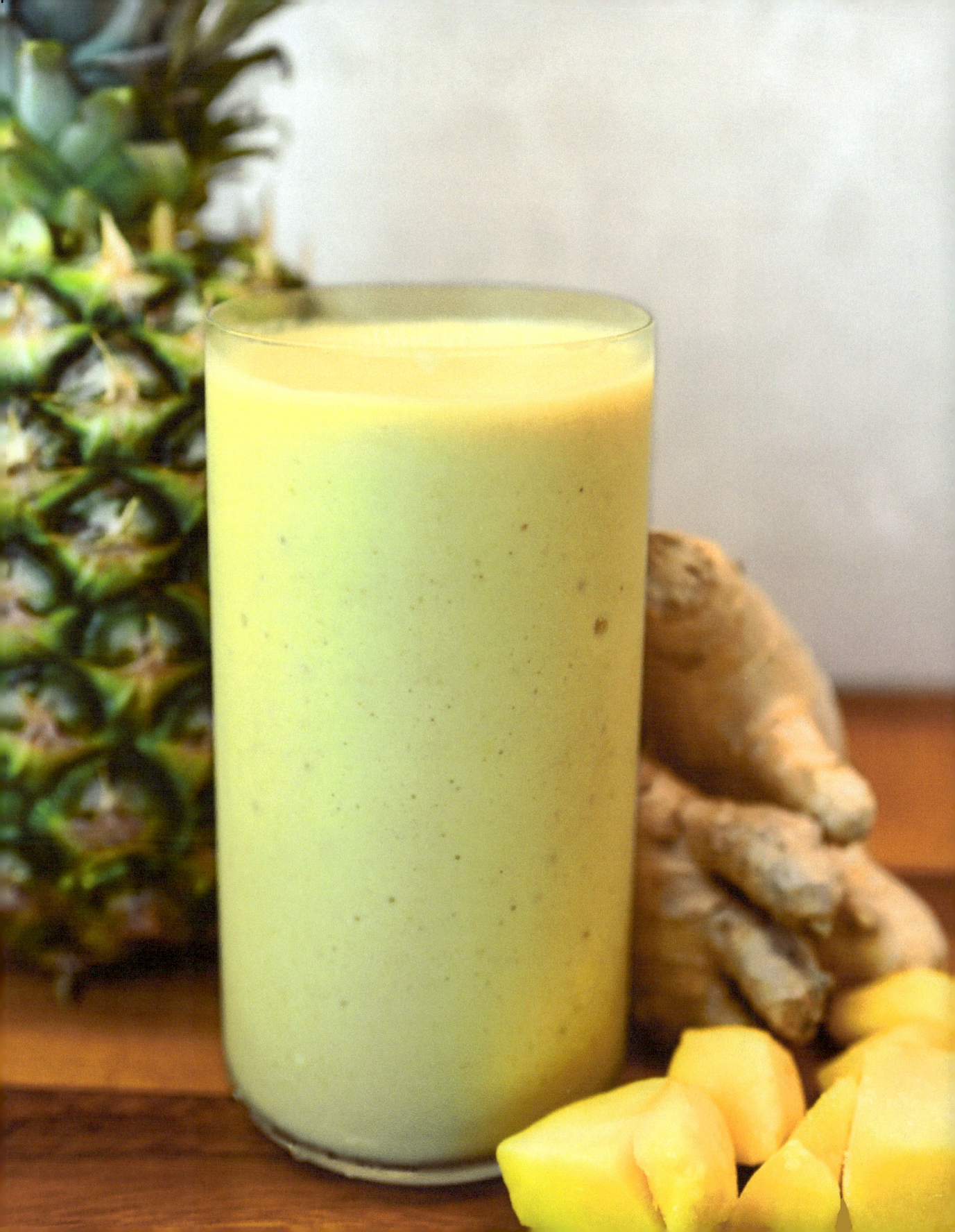

you'vegotkale

smoothie

This is by far the best smoothie for breakfast. Holly would often drink it before she opened. This one also was a difficult smoothie for new staff to learn the correct consistency of.

Ingredients

- 1 cup almond milk
- ½ cup frozen banana
- ½ cup frozen apple
- 1 large kale leaf
- 1 knob ginger
- 1 scoop hemp protein

Instructions

1. Add all the ingredients to a blender.
2. Blend until smooth and creamy.
3. Pour into a glass and enjoy immediately!

TIPS

 Cut up and freeze an apple or two to have on hand when you plan to make this. If you forget, you can add fresh apple. Just start with less milk so that your smoothie comes out the correct consistency. Always put your kale leaf on top of your frozen fruit.

 If you find it comes out too liquidy for your liking, put less almond milk in.

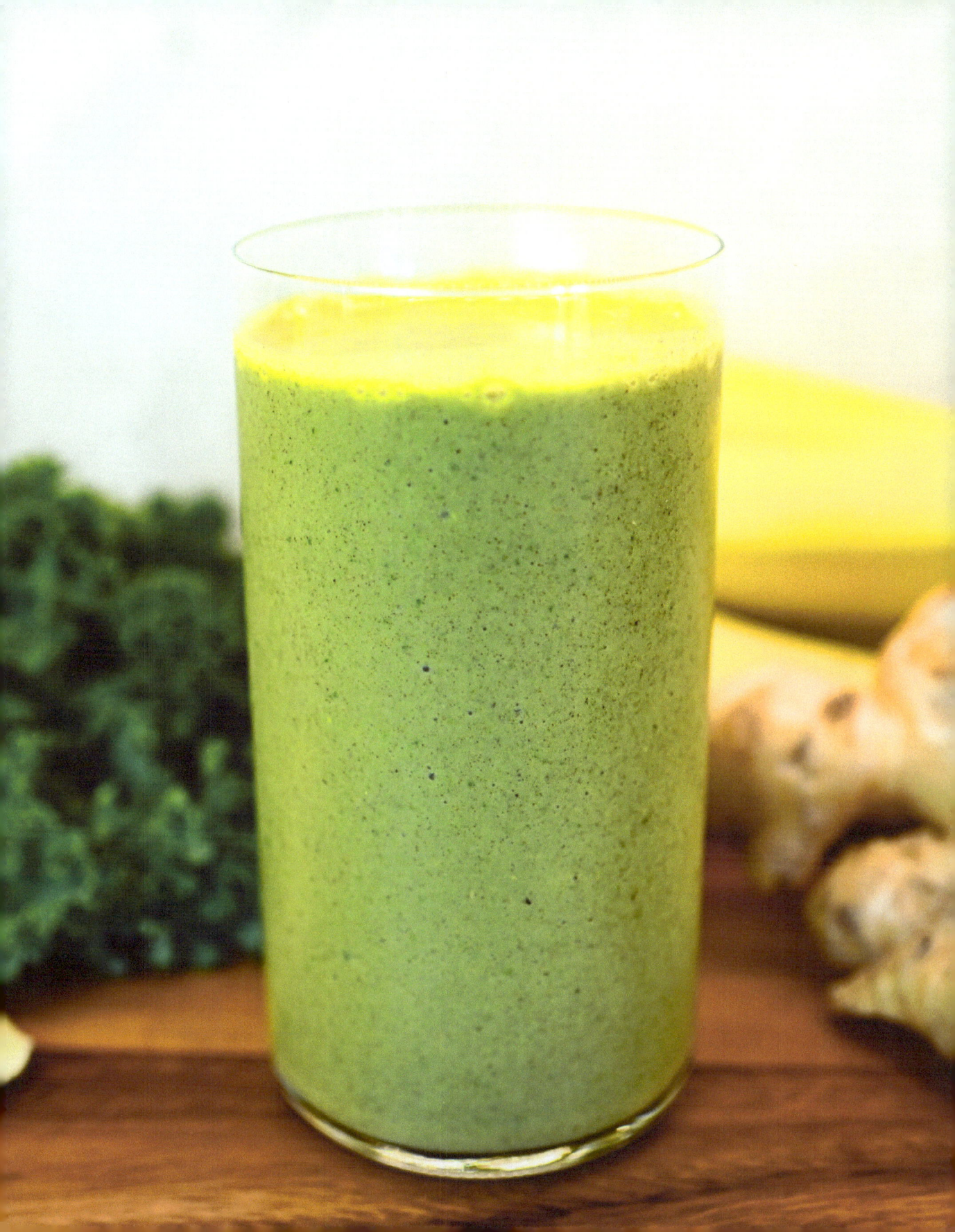

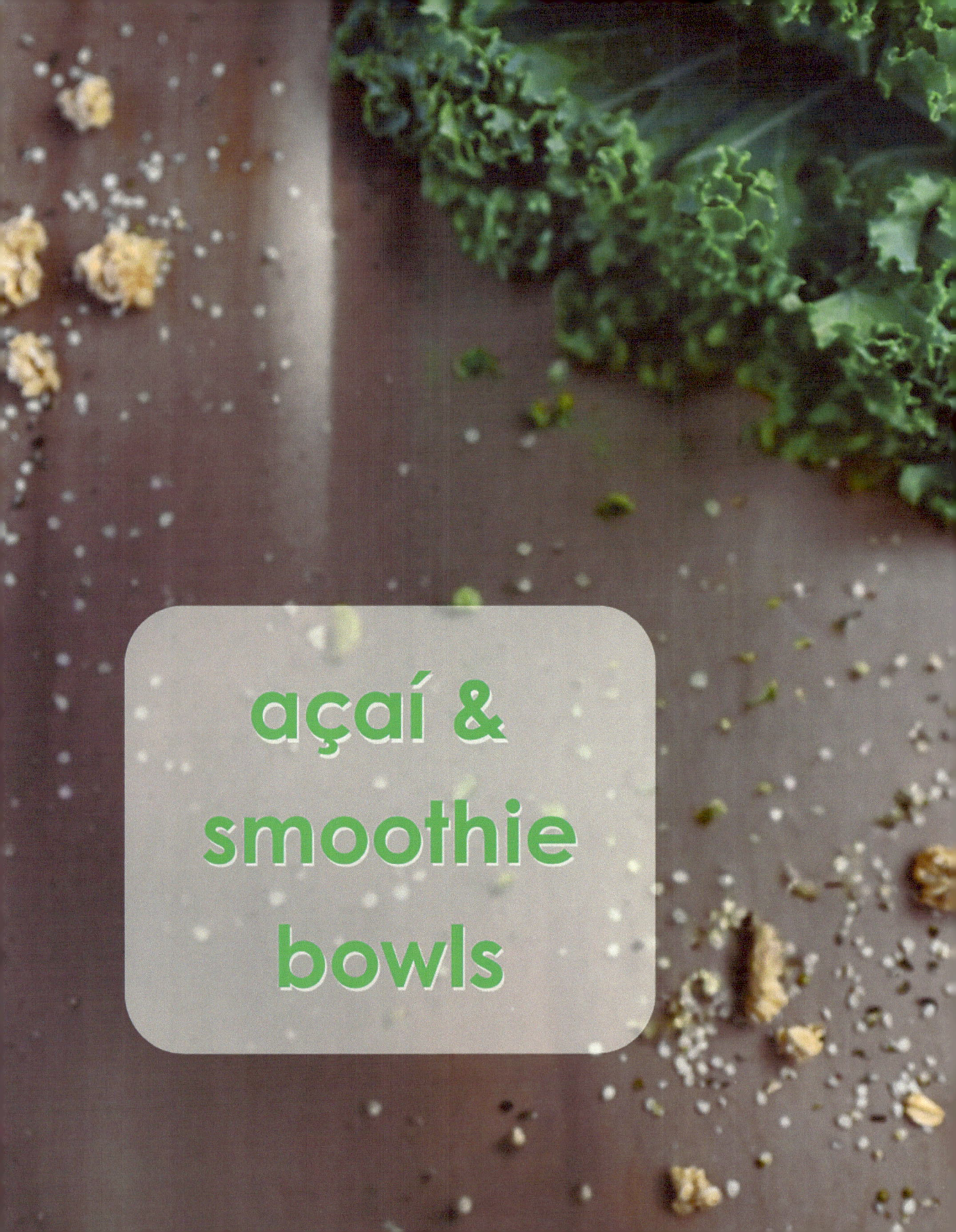

açaí & smoothie bowls

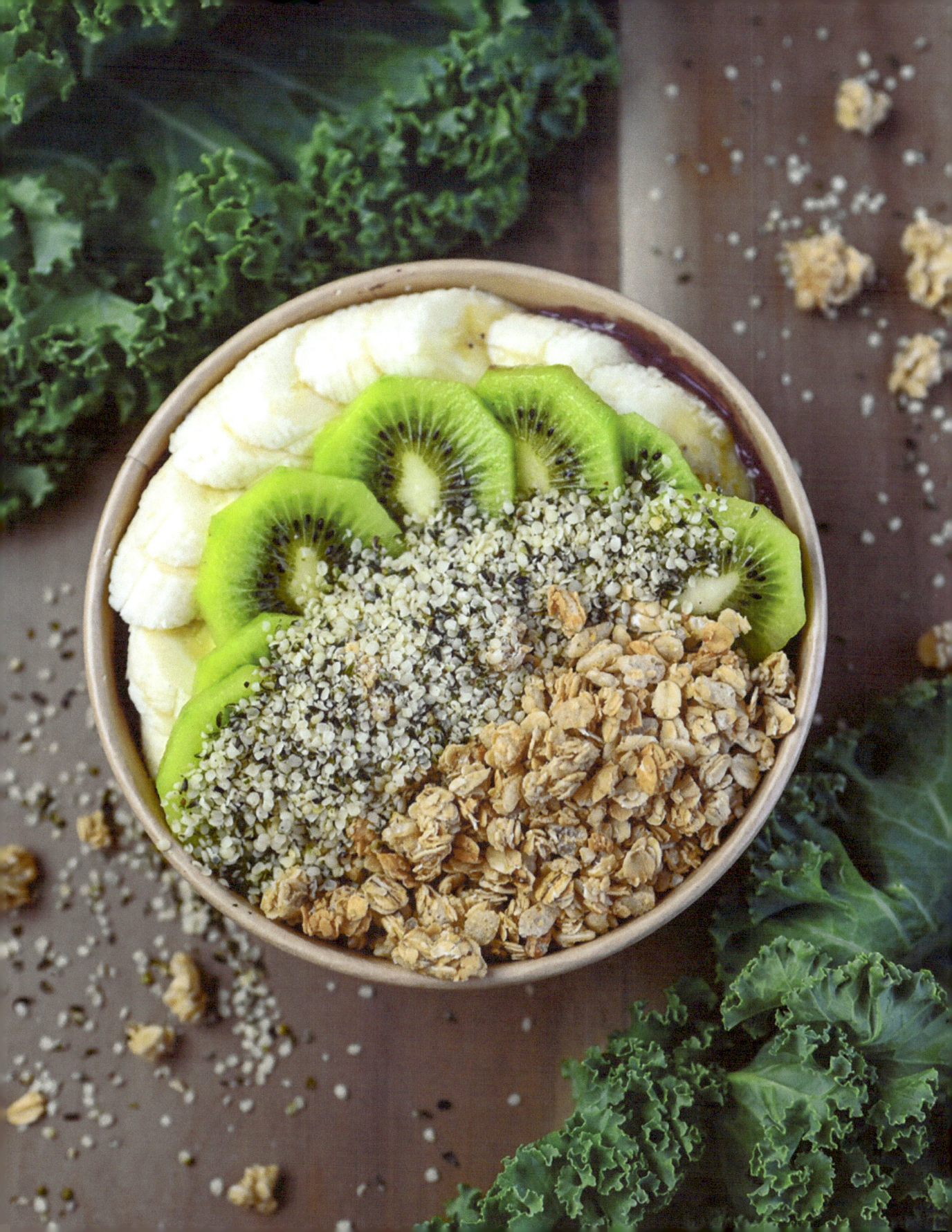

AÇAÍ & SMOOTHIE

Açaí bowls are not only pretty to look at but also a deliciously healthy way to fuel your day! The açaí berry, which comes from the rainforests of Central and South America, is packed with powerful antioxidants that may help support heart health, boost brain function, and promote overall well-being.

But that's not all—these little berries are also rich in healthy fats, fiber, and a variety of essential vitamins and minerals like potassium, calcium, and B vitamins. So, when you dig into an açaí bowl, you're not just treating your taste buds, you're giving your body a nourishing boost too!

Top it off with your favorite toppings, and you've got a tasty, energizing snack or meal that's as good for you as it is beautiful. What's not to love about that?

Little Apple's Café's reputation for elite açaí & smoothie bowls was well-established, drawing in customers from various locations who were eager to experience the renowned dish they had seen on Instagram. This social media platform served as a powerful tool for showcasing the café's offerings, creating a visual appetite and desire among the audience.

The act of customers presenting a picture to order captures the essence of modern dining trends, where visual appeal on digital platforms can significantly boost a restaurant's popularity and customer engagement. The café's ability to deliver on these expectations not only satisfied the immediate cravings but also reinforced its status as a destination for high-quality, visually appealing culinary creations.

To make an açaí bowl, start by selecting high quality unsweetened açaí. Holly prefers using frozen bricks or cubes; her go to is Tambor Açaí. If you plan to use another brand or puree, you may have to adjust the amount of liquid depending on what consistency you like for your bowls. Little Apple's açaí bowls are known for their firm consistency, which makes for a good placeholder to secure your toppings.

BOWL INSTRUCTIONS

Start by breaking your frozen açaí brick into chunks and put in the blender. Then, you will add your other frozen fruit and items the recipe calls for. Last, you will add your liquid. 4oz is standard if your frozen items are solid. If in doubt, start with less liquid, you can always add more. Once you have a smooth and thick base, use a spatula, scoop it into a bowl, and add your favorite toppings. The key is to achieve a balance of textures and flavors that not only delight the palate but also provide a nutritious meal or snack.

The process is the same to make smoothie bowls, except you would use all frozen fruit and no açaí.

TIP

 If you are do not want bananas in your acai bowl, try substituting frozen blueberries. You will need to add more liquid to get the correct consistency. Start out with 5 ounces and if it is not blending, add a little bit more until you achieve the desired consistency.

QUICK INSTRUCTIONS

GUIDE TO MAKING AN AÇAÍ & SMOOTHIE BOWLS:

- Select high-quality, unsweetened frozen açaí bricks or cubes.
- Break the açaí into chunks and place in a blender.
- Add other frozen fruits and ingredients as per your recipe.
- Pour in 4 ounces of liquid if using solid frozen items; adjust as needed for desired consistency.
- Blend until you achieve a smooth, thick base.
- Scoop into a bowl with a spatula.
- Garnish with your choice of toppings, aiming for a mix of textures and flavors.
- For a smoothie bowl, simply use a variety of frozen fruits without açaí.

REMEMBER

 The goal is to create a delicious and nutritious treat that satisfies both taste and health. Enjoy your homemade açaí & smoothie bowl!

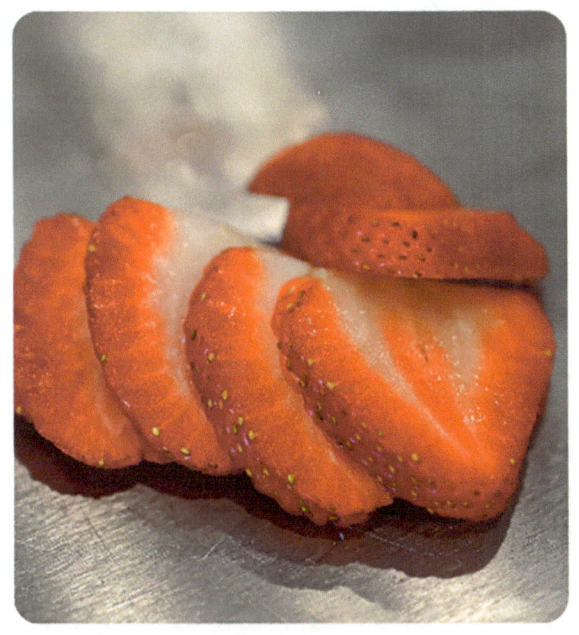

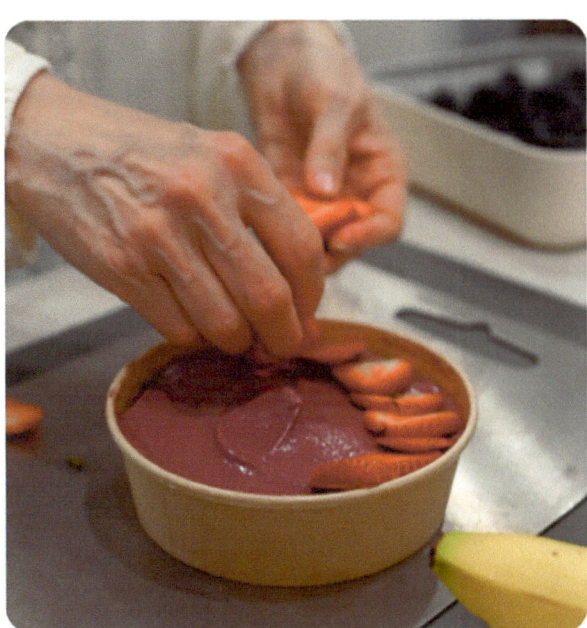

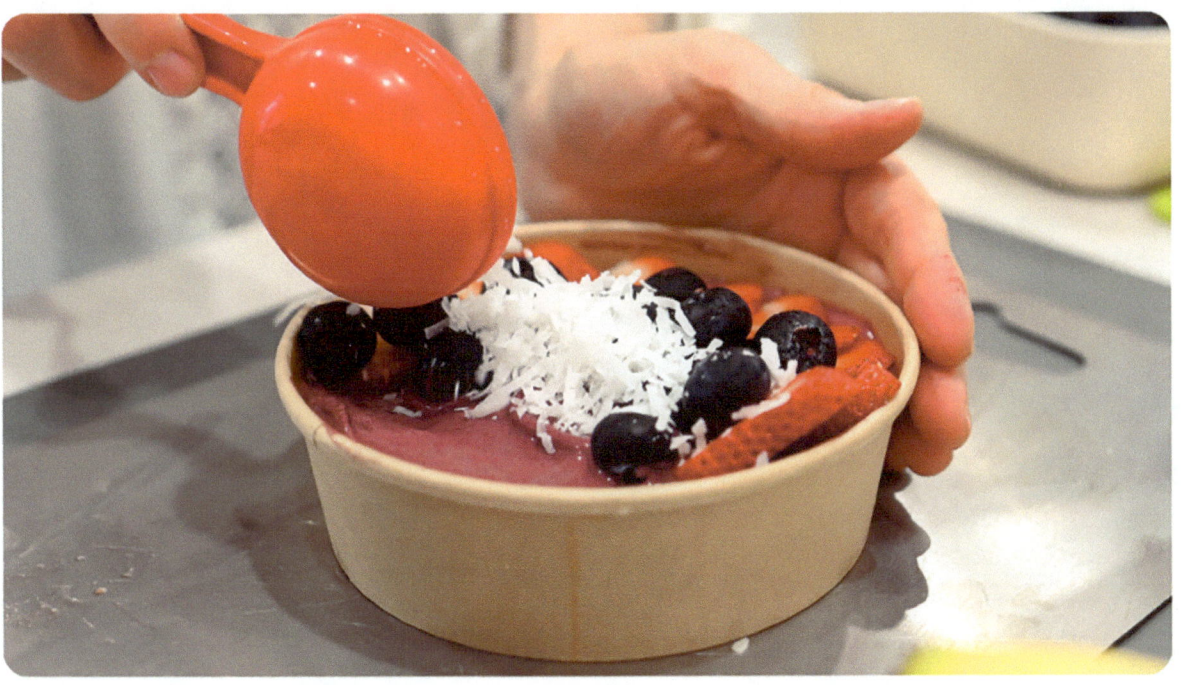

almondjoy

açaí bowl

Ingredients

This was the number one selling açaí bowl of all time. The staff would often try to guess at the end of each month how many we sold.

Base:

Blend together:

- 1 brick (5 ounces) açaí
- 1.5 cups frozen bananas
- 1 tablespoon almond butter
- 4 ounces almond milk

Toppings:

- 1 large strawberry, sliced
- 2 ounces blueberries
- 2 ounces coconut flakes
- 4 ounces granola
- 1 teaspoon bee pollen

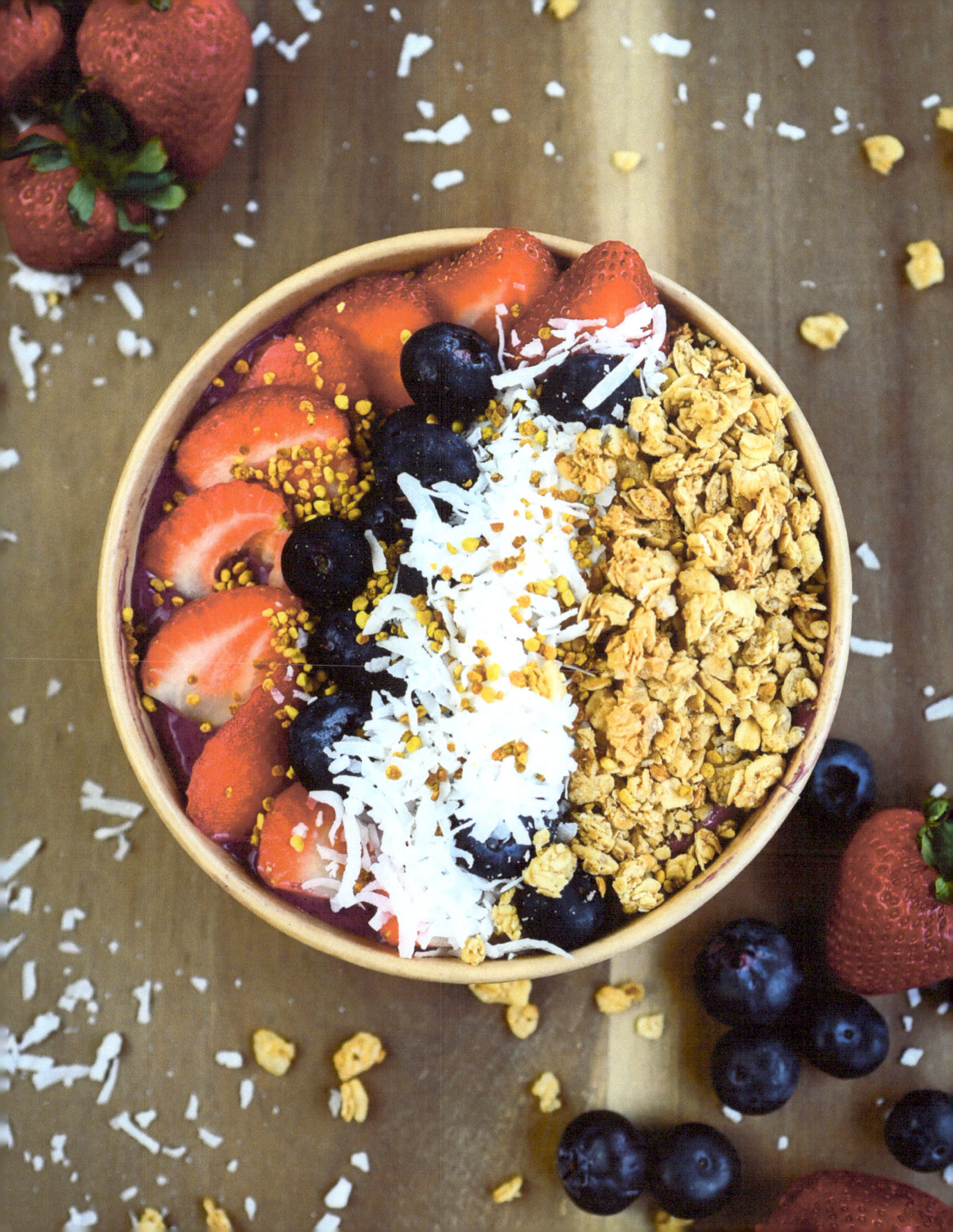

amazonaçaí

Ingredients

Base:

Blend together:

- 1 brick (5 ounces) açaí
- 7 ounces pineapple
- 1 cup frozen banana
- 4 ounces coconut water

Toppings:

- 1 banana, sliced
- 2 ounces pineapple, sliced
- 2 ounces coconut flakes
- 4 ounces granola
- 2 ounces hemp seeds

Holly made this bowl for a famous person everyday one summer while they were filming in town. It is also the most refreshing açaí bowl and the hardest one to blend.

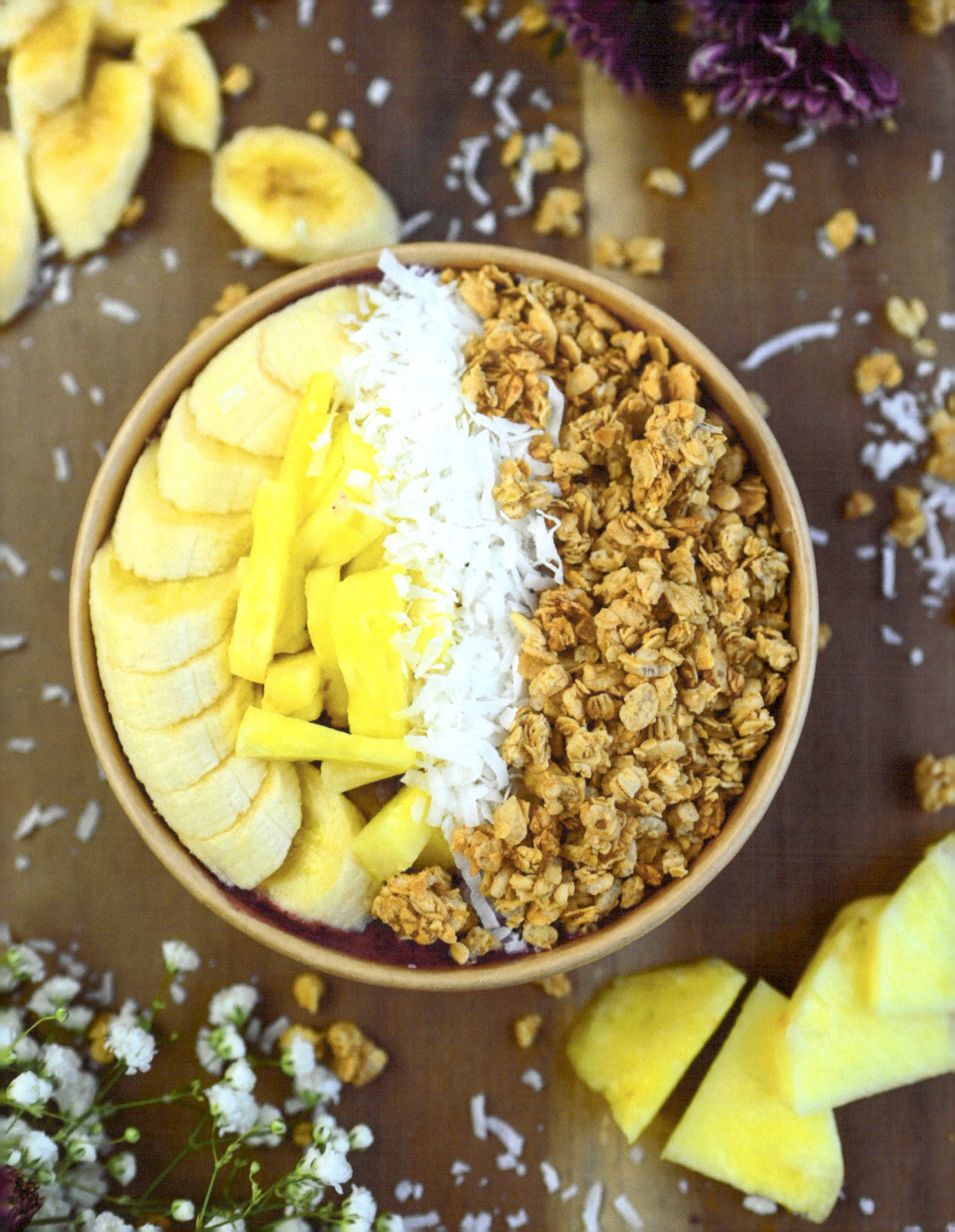

greenpeace

açaí bowl

Ingredients

Base:

Blend together:

- 1 brick (5 ounces) açaí
- 1.5 cups frozen bananas
- 1 medium piece of kale
- 4 ounces almond milk

Toppings:

- 1 banana, sliced
- 1 kiwi, sliced
- 2 ounces hempseeds
- 4 ounces granola

The greenpeace is so peaceful, smooth and tasty, you'd never guess there's kale hiding in it!

TIP

 Sub sliced almonds in place of the granola

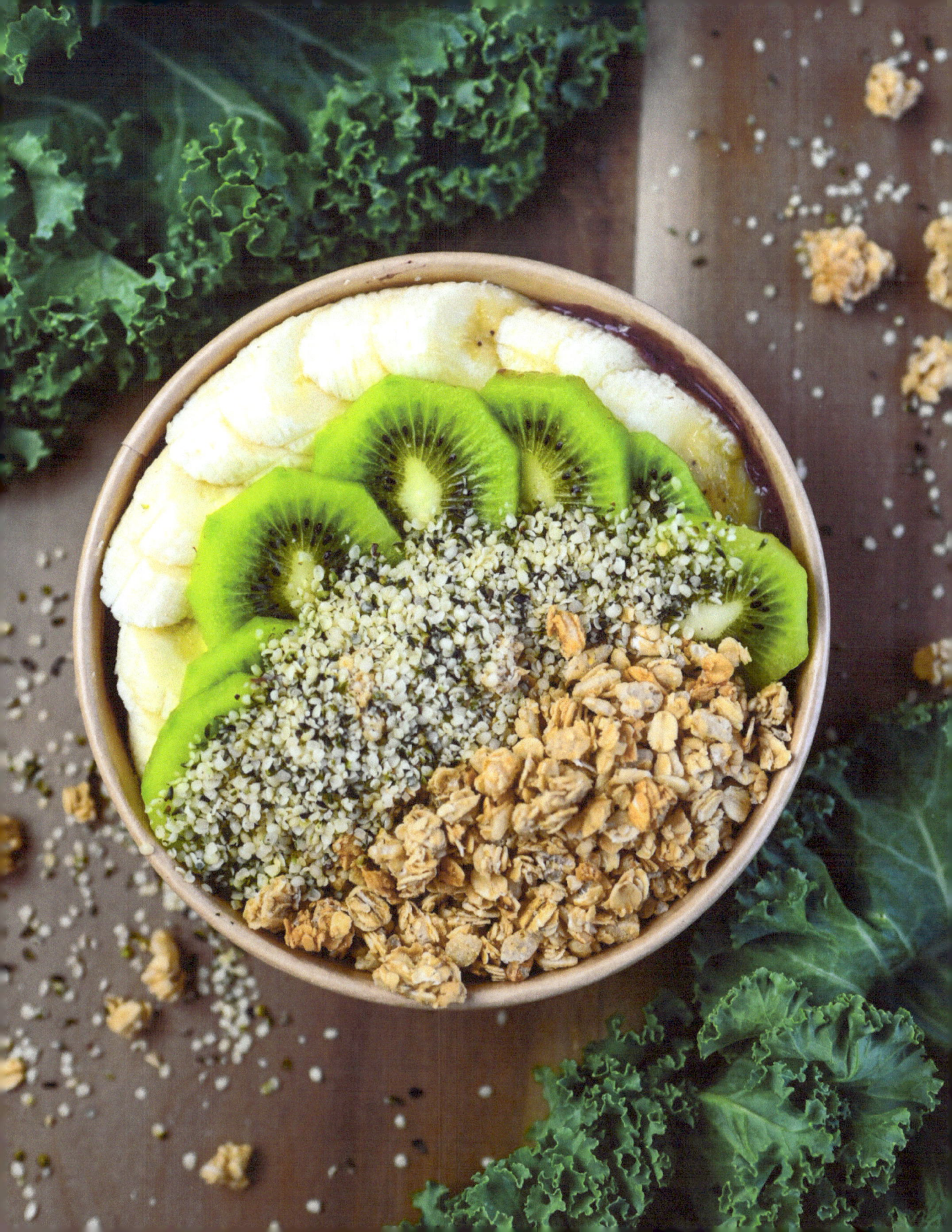

littlewarrior

Ingredients

The bowl so crave-worthy, one bite and you'll forget every other option even exists.

Base:

Blend together:

- 1 brick (5 ounces) açaí
- 1.5 cups frozen bananas
- 1 tablespoon peanut butter
- 4 ounces almond milk

Toppings:

- 3 large strawberries, sliced
- 2 ounces peanuts
- 4 ounces granola
- 1 tablespoon peanut butter on top

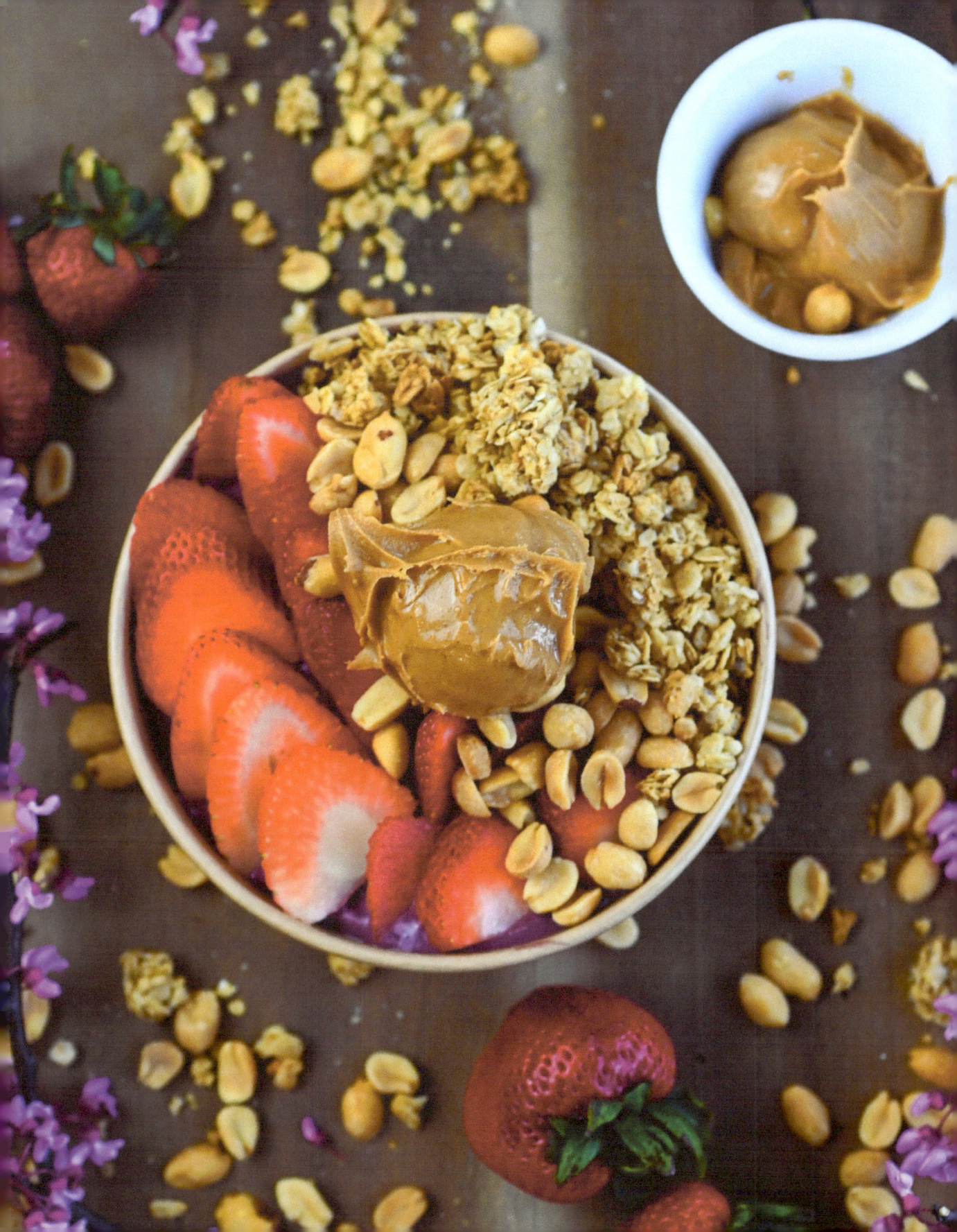

peanutbutter&jealous

smoothie bowl

One of our beloved customers travels great lengths for his peanutbutter&jealous fix.

Ingredients

Base:

Blend together:

- 2.5 cups frozen bananas
- 4 ounces almond milk
- 1 ounce peanut butter
- 1 teaspoon raw cacao

Toppings:

- 1 banana, sliced
- 2 ounces cacao nibs
- 2 ounces peanuts
- 2 ounces granola
- 1 ounce peanut butter on top

TIPS

 Pairs well with chocolate or vanilla protein

 This bowl was the hardest for new staff members to master. If you put your banana topping on and it sinks into the base, it's too soft.

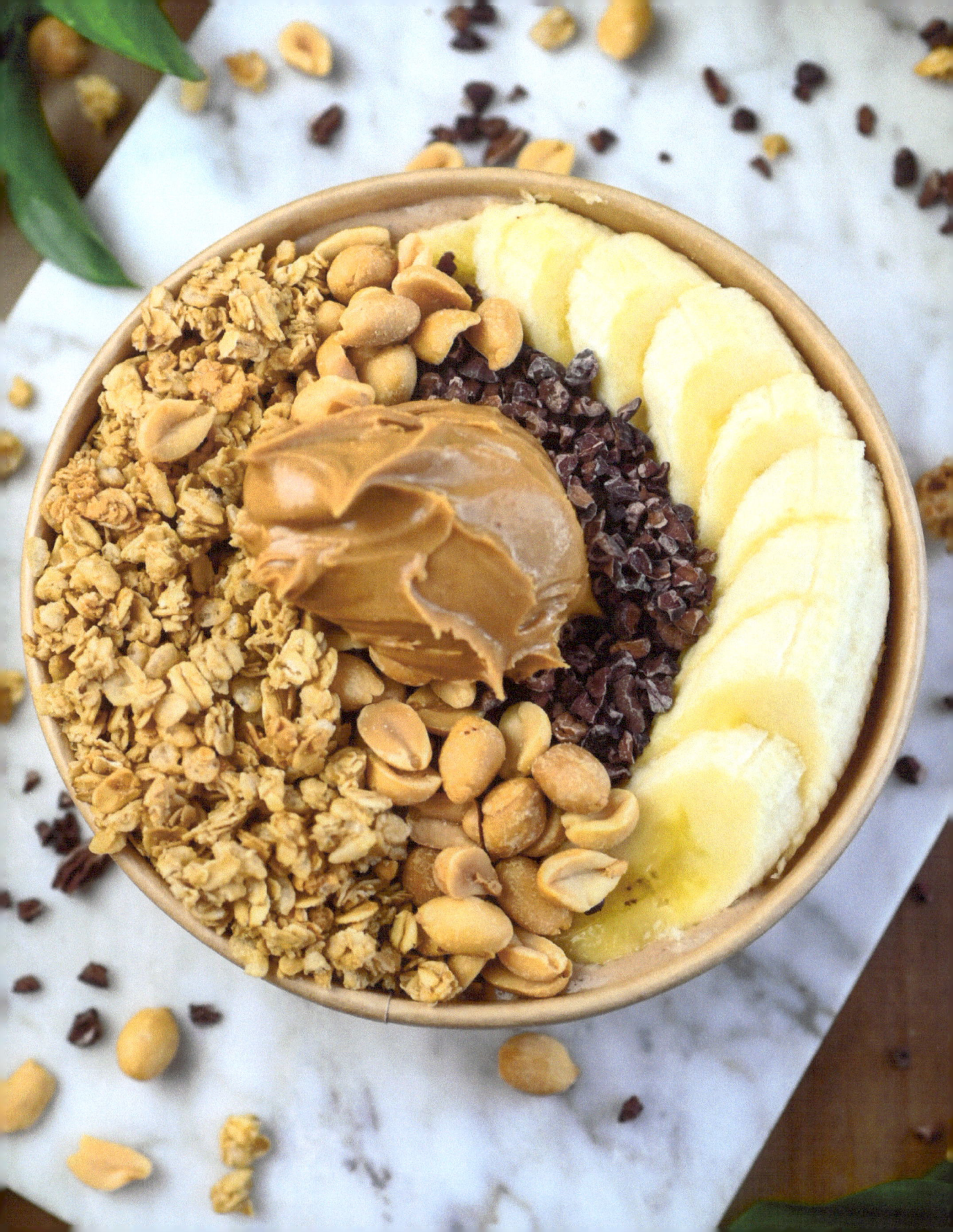

pinksunset

smoothie bowl

Ingredients

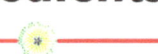

The pinksunset was the most popular smoothie bowl.

Base:

Blend together:

- 2 cups frozen strawberries
- 1 cup frozen bananas
- 4 ounces almond milk

Toppings:

- 1 banana, sliced
- 1 large strawberry, sliced
- 4 ounces coconut flakes
- 4 ounces granola
- 1 ounce peanut butter on top

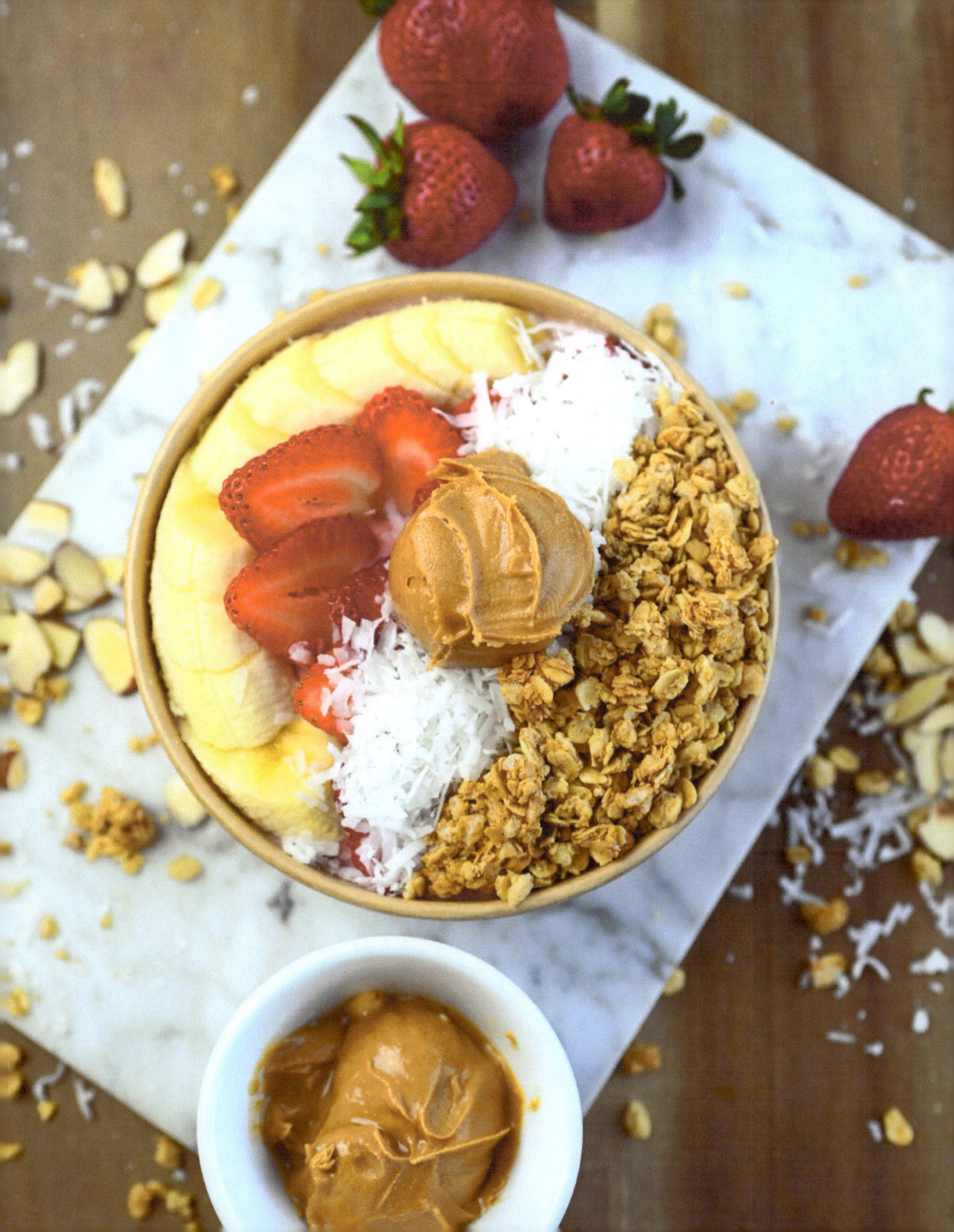

rise&shine

smoothie bowl

rise&shine tastes like a party in your mouth.

Ingredients

Base:

Blend together:

- 1 cup frozen pineapples
- 1 cup frozen mangos
- ½ cup frozen bananas
- 4 ounces coconut milk

Toppings:

- 1 kiwi
- 4 ounces pineapples
- 4 ounces coconut flakes
- 4 ounces granola

TIP

 Pairs well with vanilla protein

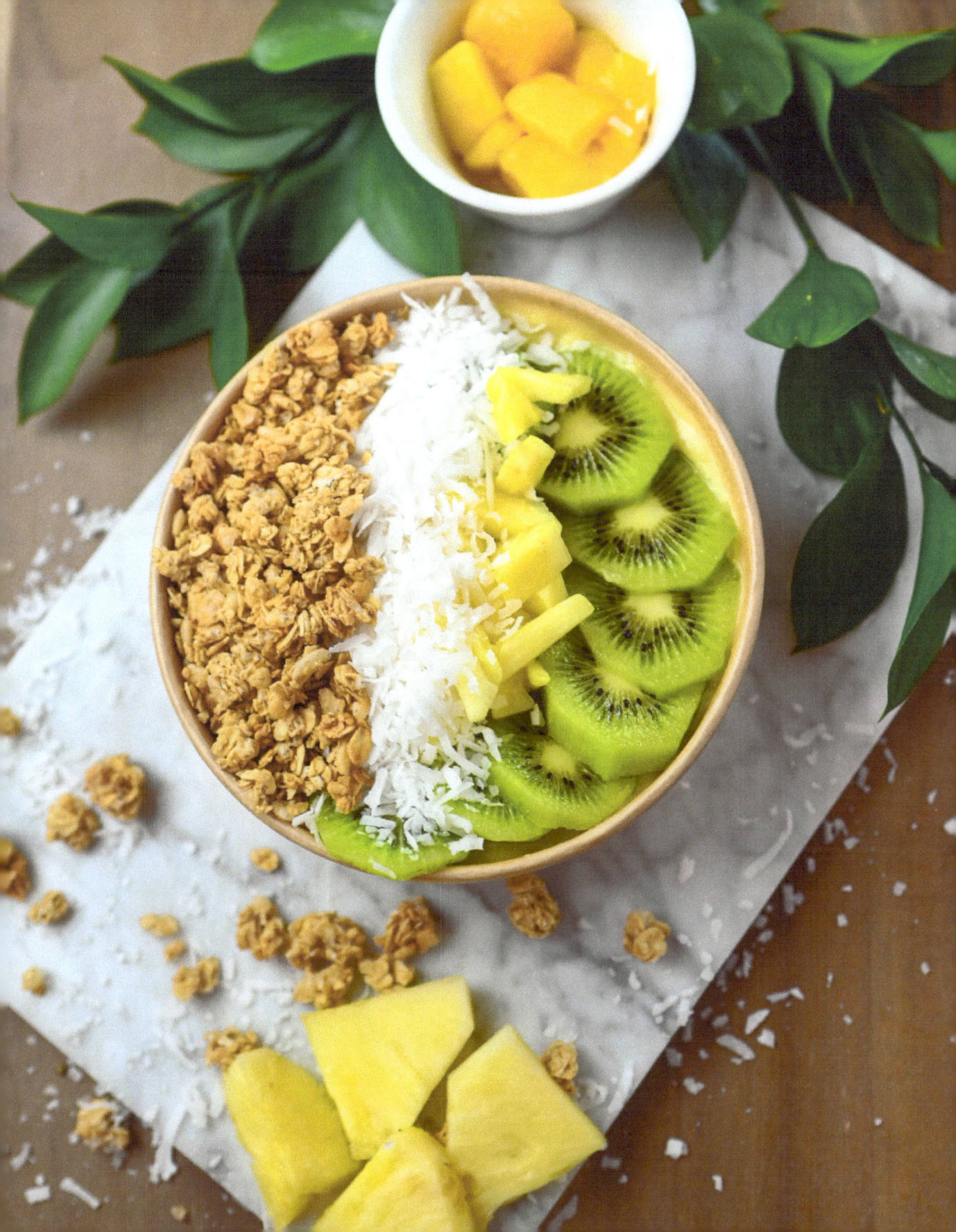

the**unicorn**

smoothie bowl

Ingredients

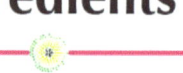

Base:

Blend together:

- 1 cup frozen pitayas
- ⅓ cup frozen bananas
- ⅓ cup frozen mango
- 1 tablespoon honey
- 4 ounces coconut water

Toppings:

- 3 medium strawberries, sliced
- 2 ounces coconut flakes
- 4 ounces sliced almonds

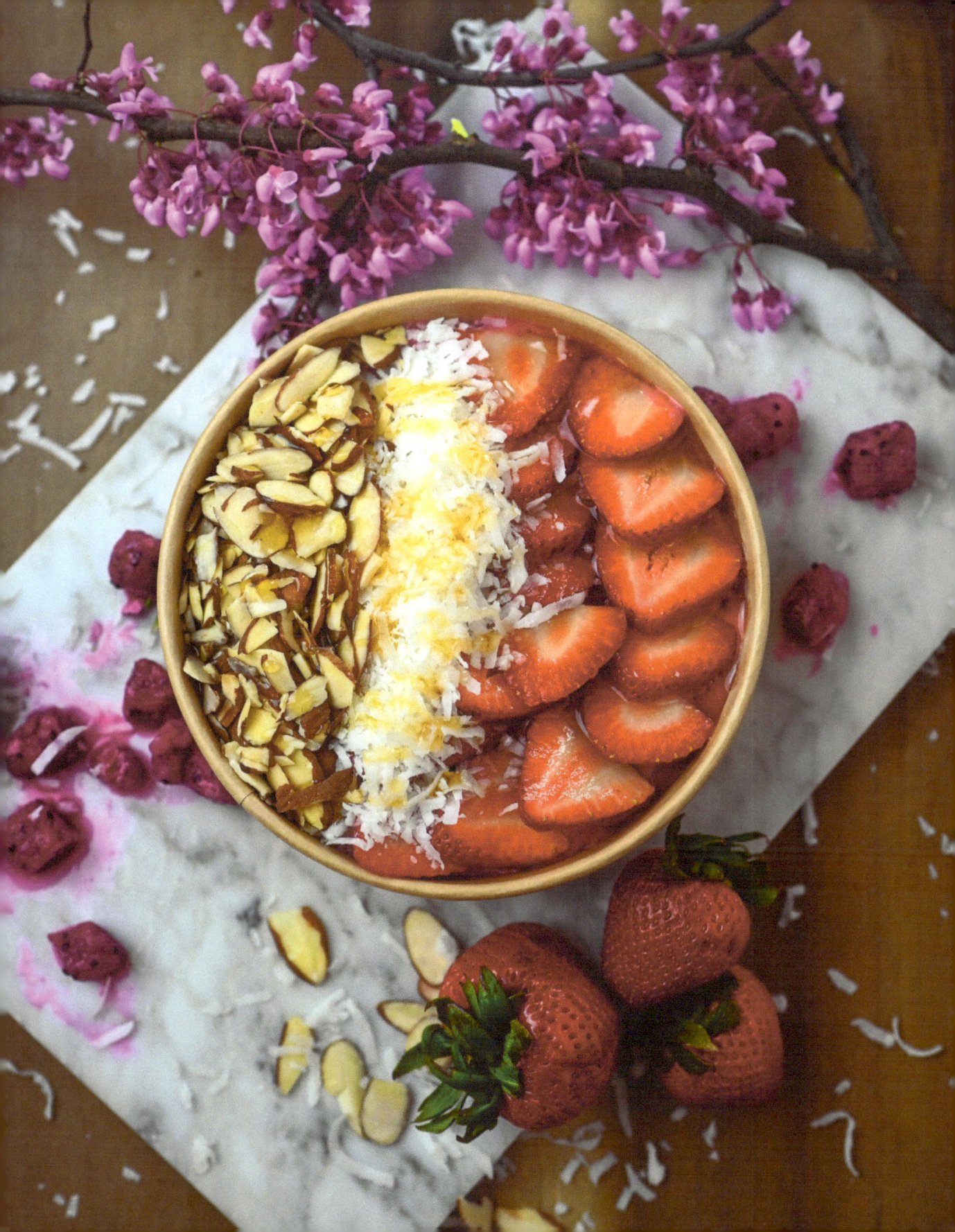

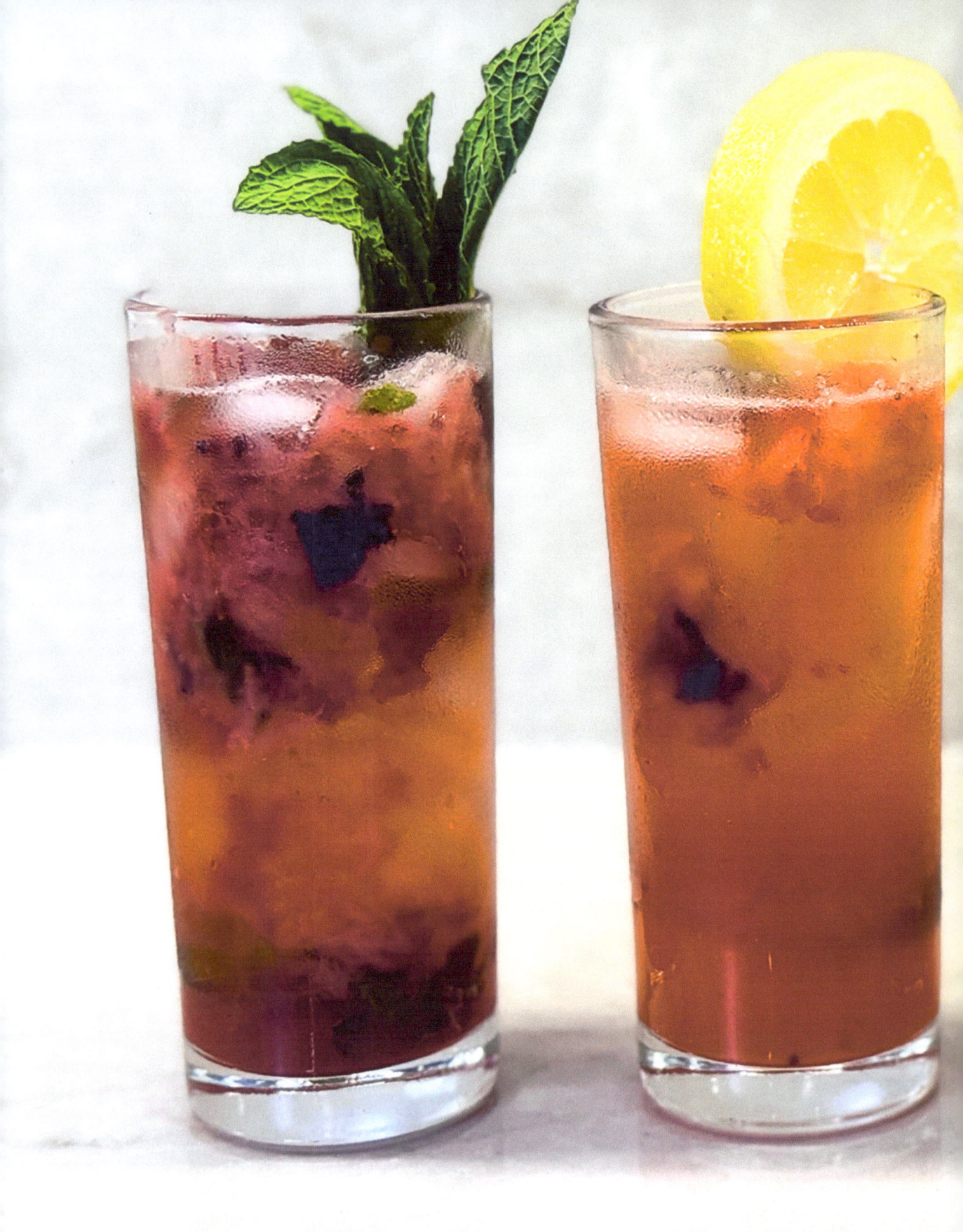

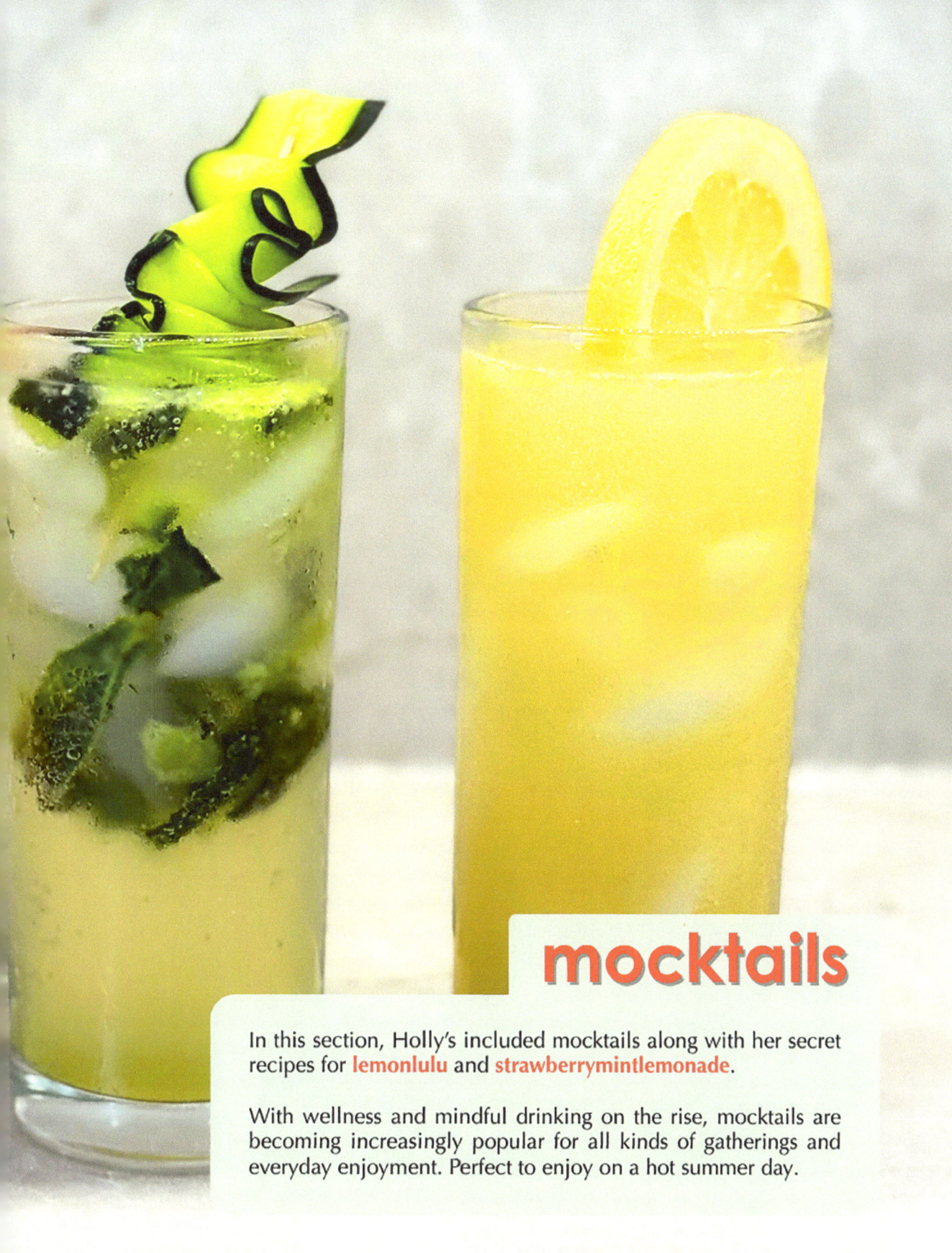

mocktails

In this section, Holly's included mocktails along with her secret recipes for lemonlulu and strawberrymintlemonade.

With wellness and mindful drinking on the rise, mocktails are becoming increasingly popular for all kinds of gatherings and everyday enjoyment. Perfect to enjoy on a hot summer day.

MOCKTAILS

Mocktails, the non-alcoholic version of cocktails, are indeed gaining popularity for their delicious taste and potential health benefits. They offer a refreshing alternative to alcoholic drinks, often incorporating a variety of fruits, herbs, and spices that not only tantalize the taste buds but also contribute to a healthier lifestyle. For instance, using ingredients like fresh mint, ginger, or citrus fruits can add a burst of flavor as well as a dose of vitamins and antioxidants.

Mocktails can be a smart choice for those looking to reduce calorie intake, as they can be crafted with less sugar and empty calories compared to many alcoholic beverages. They're a fantastic way to enjoy a sophisticated drink without the negative effects of alcohol, such as hangovers or addiction risks. Whether it's a sparkling berry spritzer or a ginger lemon fizz, mocktails are a trendy, tasty, and wholesome addition to any gathering or a cozy night in.

To whip up a delightful mocktail, you'll need a few essential tools to mix, muddle, and measure your ingredients to perfection. Start with a sturdy cocktail shaker, which is key for combining your juices, syrups, and other mix-ins thoroughly. A muddler will be your best friend for crushing herbs and fruits to release their full flavors, while a jigger ensures you're pouring the right amounts to keep your mocktail's taste balanced. Don't forget a long-handled bar spoon for stirring and a strainer to achieve that smooth, professional finish. As for the mocktail itself, let your creativity flow! Combine fresh juices, fizzy sodas, and a dash of sweetener, like simple syrup or agave syrup. Garnish with fresh fruit or a sprig of mint, and voilà, you have a refreshing, non-alcoholic treat that's perfect for any occasion.

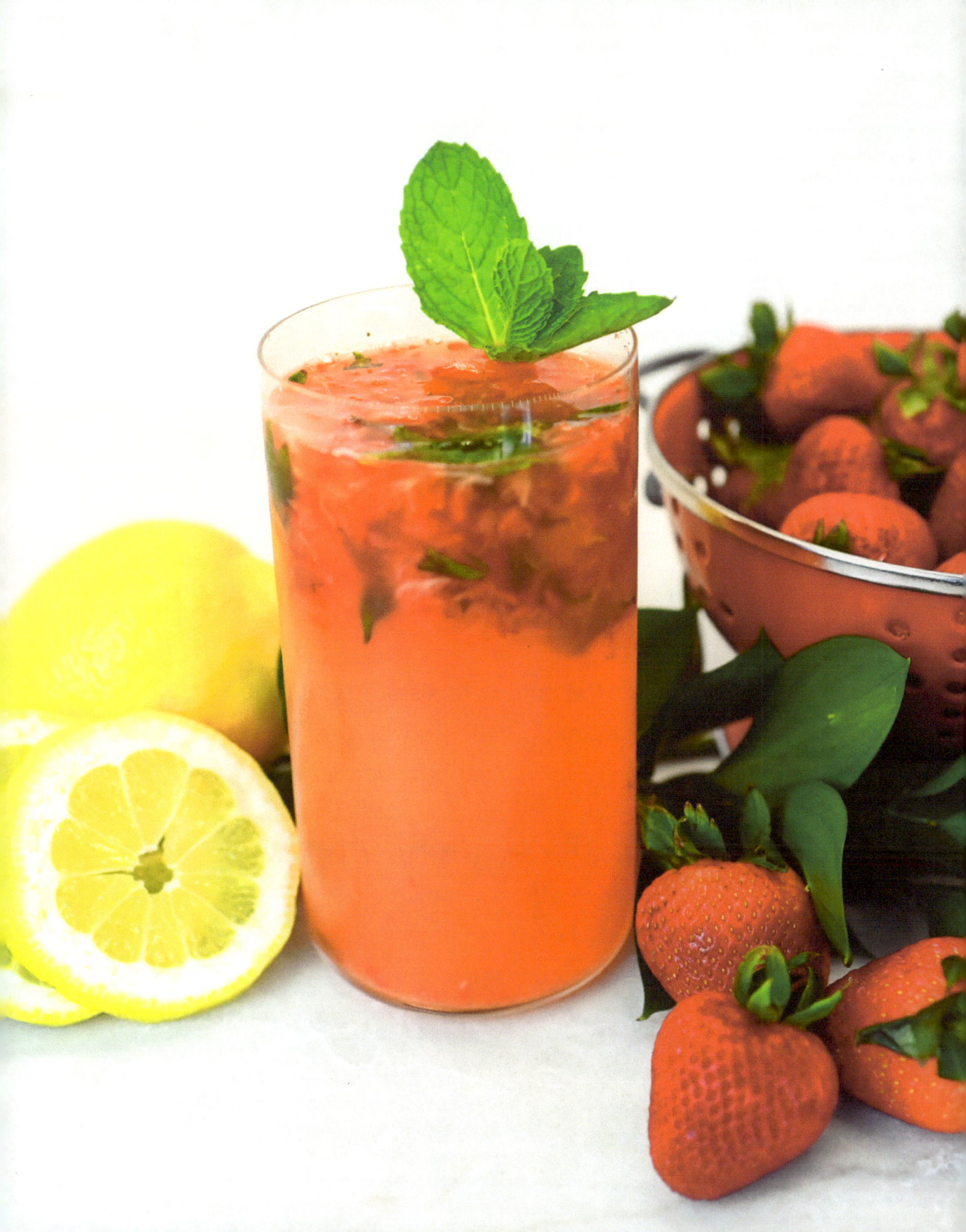

berry**fojito**

mocktail

Ingredients

- 2 strawberries
- 4 blueberries
- 6 mint leaves
- 1 teaspoon agave syrup
- 8 ounces of seltzer
- garnished with mint sprig

Instructions

- In the bottom of a sturdy glass, shaker cup or jar, muddle the strawberries, blueberries, and mint leaves until the berries are juicy and the mint is fragrant.
- Add the agave syrup, and stir to mix.
- Fill the glass with ice.
- Slowly pour in the sparkling seltzer, then gently stir to combine.
- Garnish with a fresh mint sprig, and serve immediately.

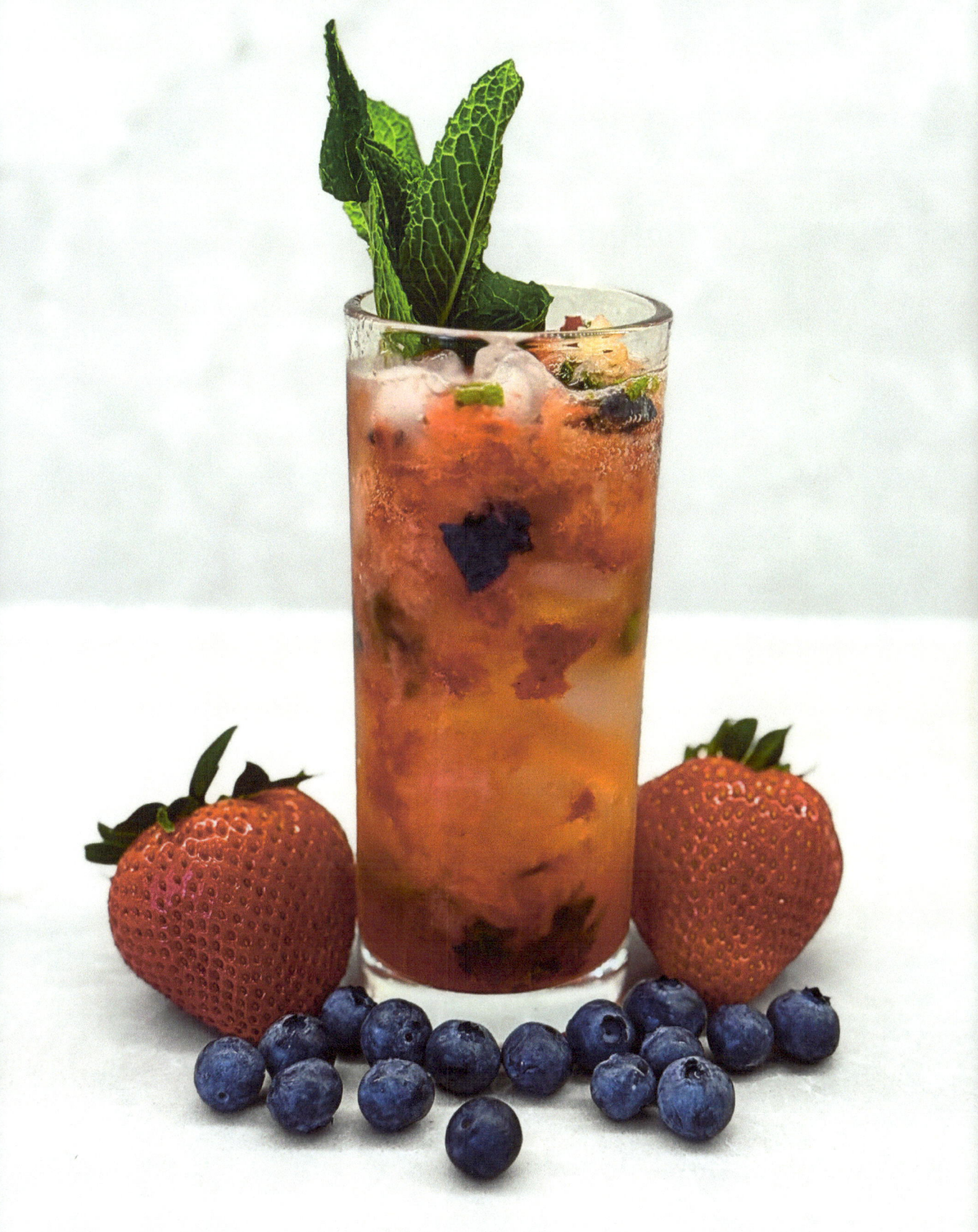

cucumber**breeze**

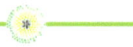

Ingredients

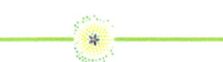

- 2 slices of cucumber
- 6 mint leaves
- 1 lime
- 1 teaspoon agave syrup
- 8 ounces of seltzer
- garnish with a cucumber slice.

Instructions

- In the bottom of a sturdy glass or jar, muddle the cucumber slices and mint leaves until fragrant and broken down.
- Add the lime juice and agave syrup, and stir well to combine.
- Fill the glass with ice.
- Slowly pour in the sparkling seltzer, and give it a gentle stir to mix the flavors without flattening the fizz.
- Garnish with a fresh cucumber slice, and enjoy right away

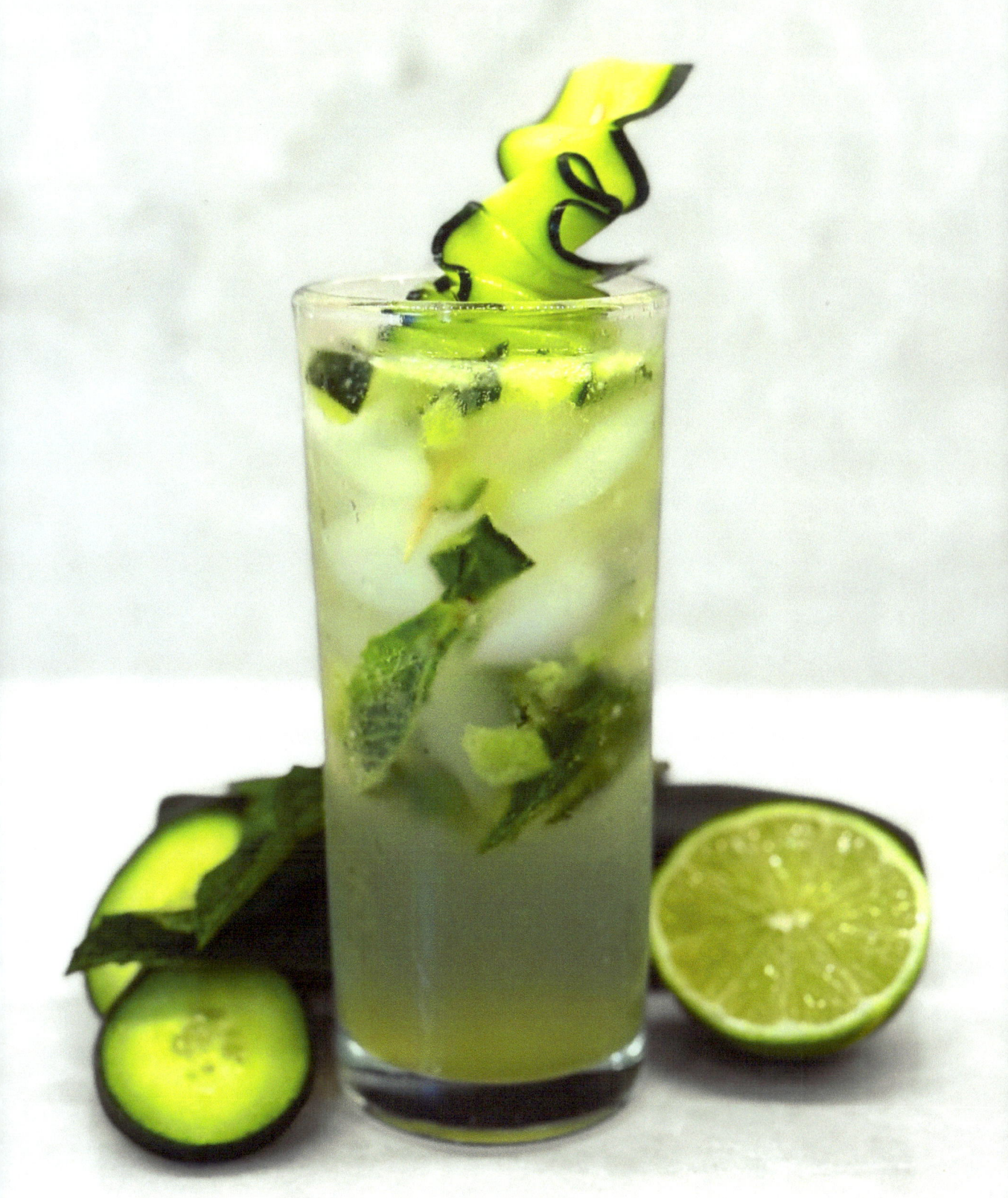

lemonberrysparkler

Ingredients

- 2 ounces fresh lemon juice
- 2 strawberries
- 4 blueberries
- 1 teaspoon agave syrup
- 8 ounces of seltzer

Instructions

- In the bottom of a sturdy glass, shaker cup or jar, muddle the strawberries and blueberries until they're well crushed and juicy.
- Add the lemon juice and agave syrup, and stir well to combine.
- Slowly pour in the sparkling seltzer, then gently stir to combine without losing the fizz.
- Garnish with a lemon wheel and enjoy immediately.

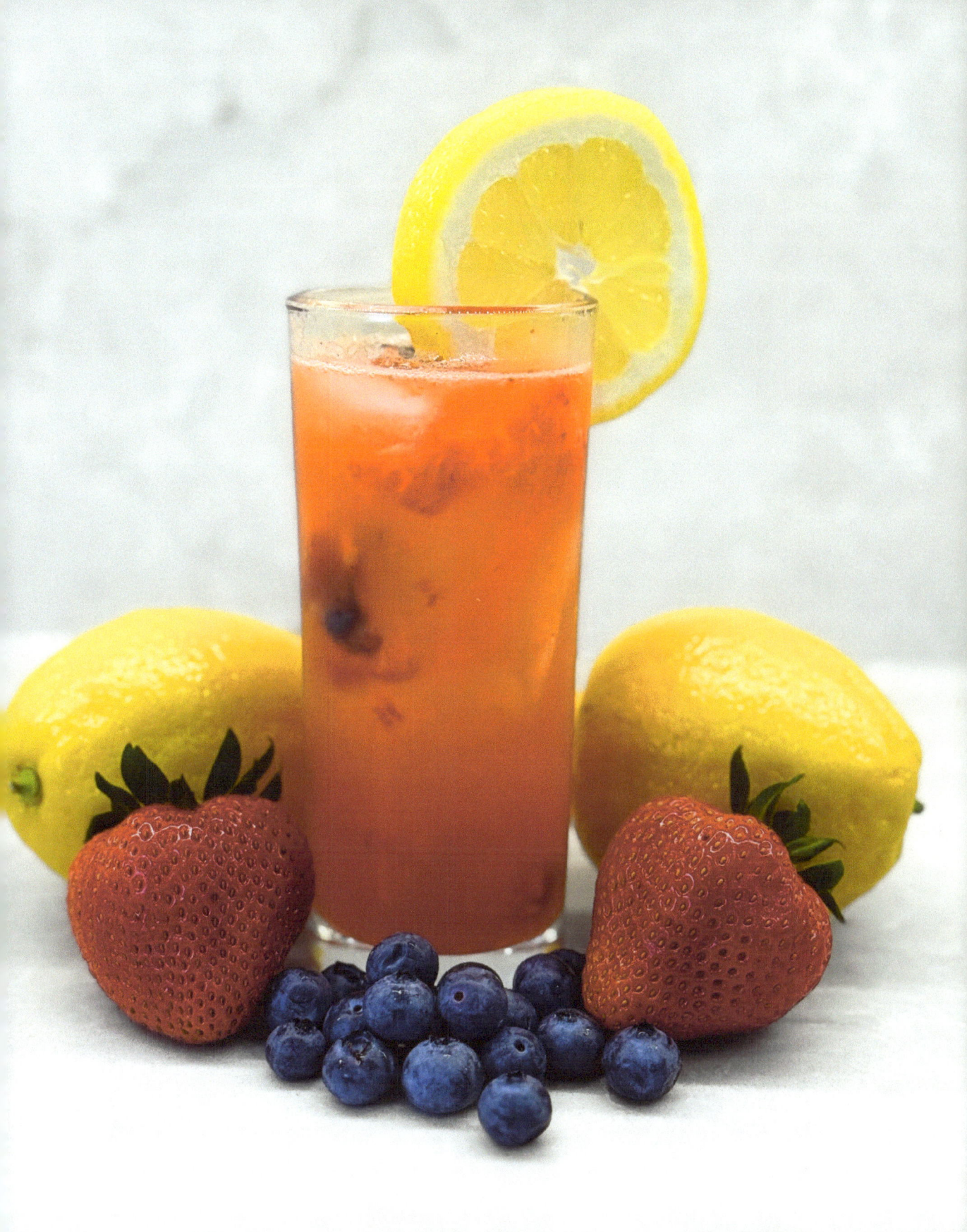

lemongingerfizz

Ingredients

- Freshly juiced:
  - 2 ounces lemon
  - 1 ounce ginger
- 1 teaspoon maple syrup
- 8 ounces of seltzer
- garnish with a lemon wheel

Instructions

- In a tall glass, shaker cup or jar, combine the lemon juice, ginger juice, and maple syrup.
- Stir well until the maple syrup is fully dissolved.
- Fill the glass with ice.
- Slowly pour in the sparkling seltzer, then gently stir to combine without losing the fizz.
- Garnish with a lemon wheel, and serve immediately.

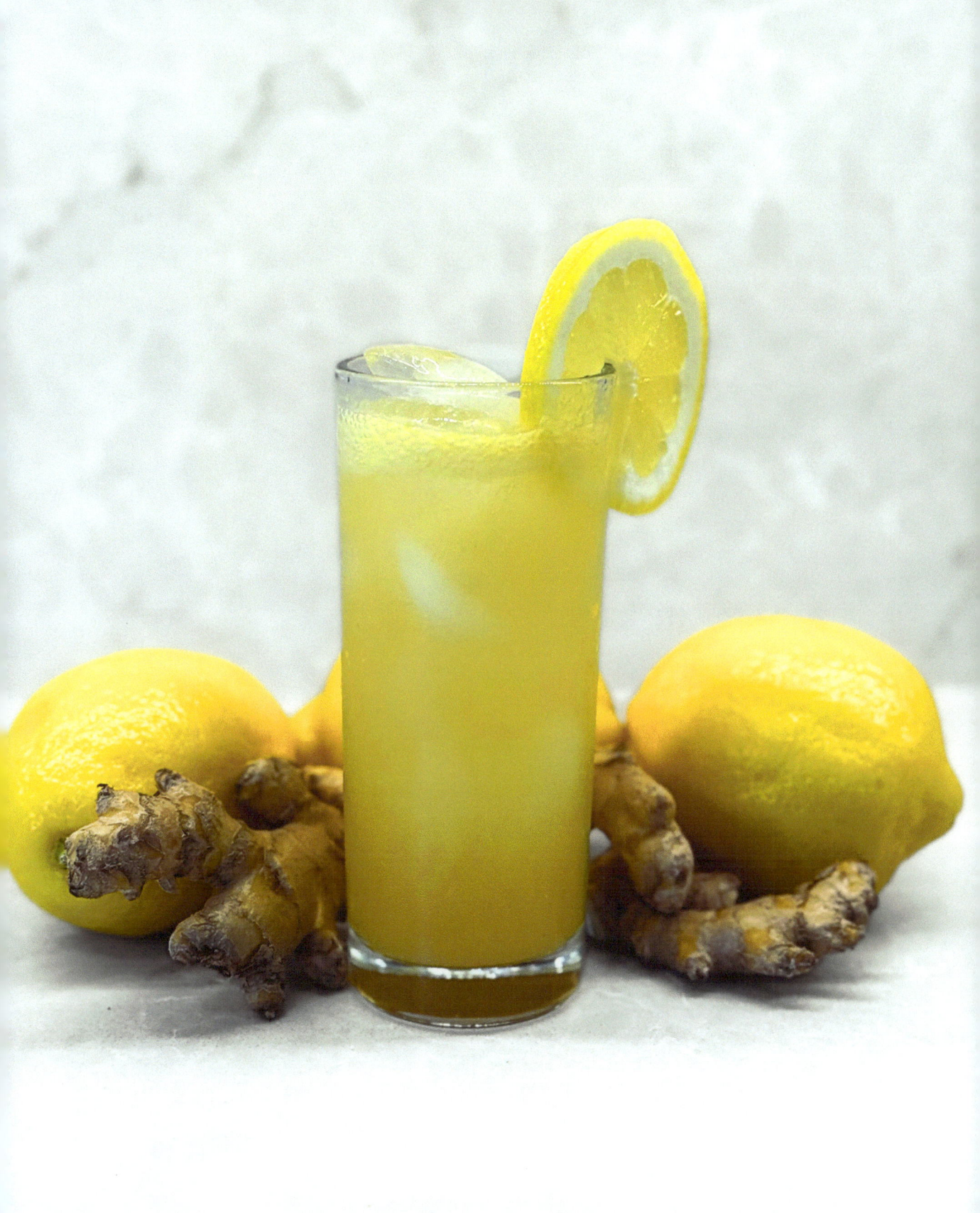

lemon*lulu*

*aka
Little Apple
Lemonade*

Ingredients

Yield 16 ounces

- 5 ounces of fresh lemon juice
- 1 teaspoon agave syrup
- 11 ounces filtered water

Instructions

- In a cocktail shaker, add lemon juice and filtered water
- Add agave syrup to taste about a 1 teaspoon, depending on desired sweetness.
- Fill the shaker with ice and shake vigorously until well-chilled.
- Fill a glass with ice, pour contents of cocktail shaker into glass. Keep any remaining ice in shaker to allow the muddled items to pour into the glass with fresh ice.

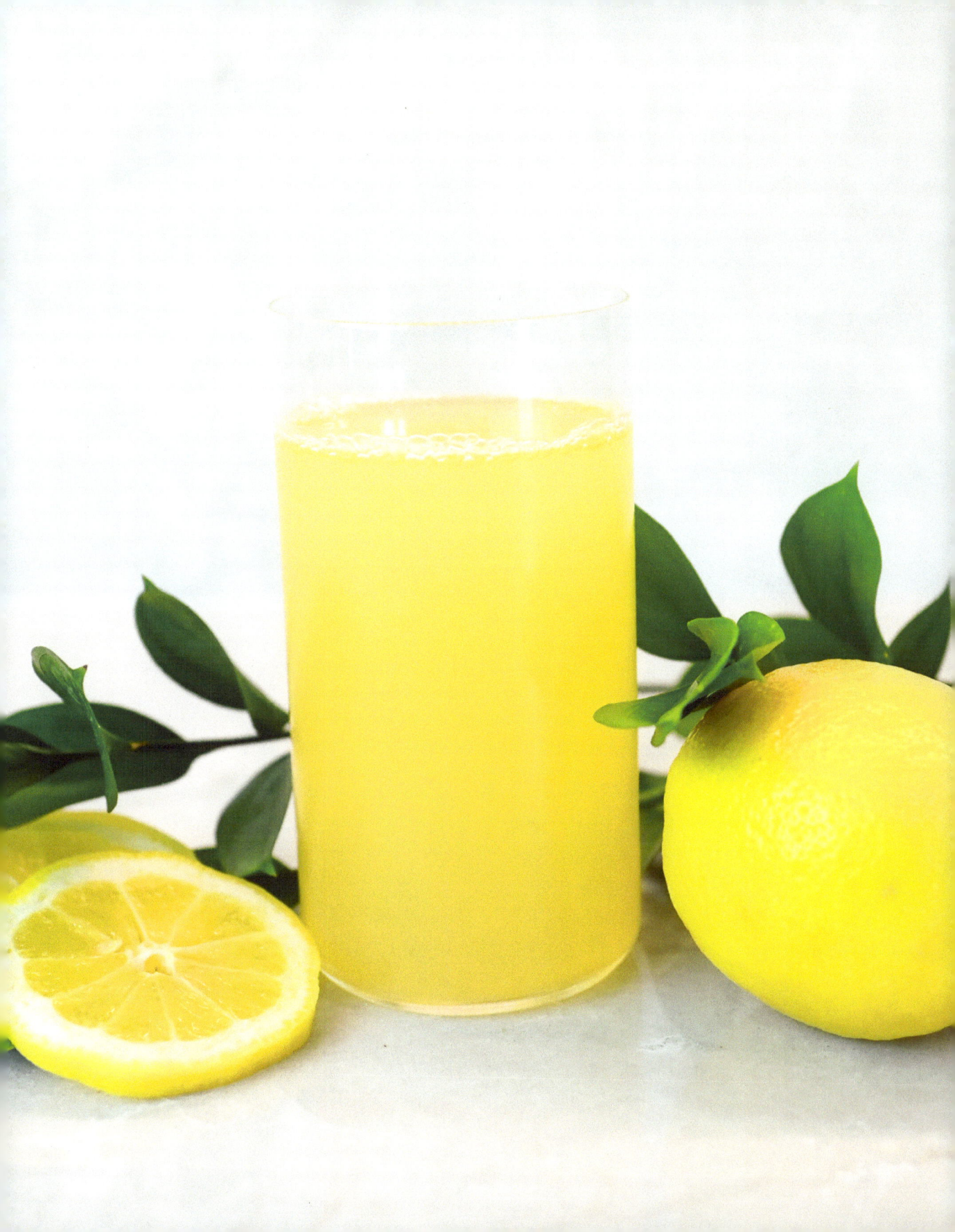

strawberrymintlemonade

mocktail

Ingredients

- 8 ounces fresh lemonade
- 2 strawberries
- 6 mint leaves
- 1 teaspoon agave syrup

Instructions

- In a cocktail shaker, muddle fresh strawberries and mint
- Add agave syrup to taste about a 1 teaspoon, depending on desired sweetness.
- Fill the shaker with ice and shake vigorously until well-chilled.
- Fill a glass with ice, pour contents of cocktail shaker into glass. Keep any remaining ice in shaker to allow the muddled items to pour into the glass with fresh ice.
- Top off with lemonade
- Garnish with a sprig of mint

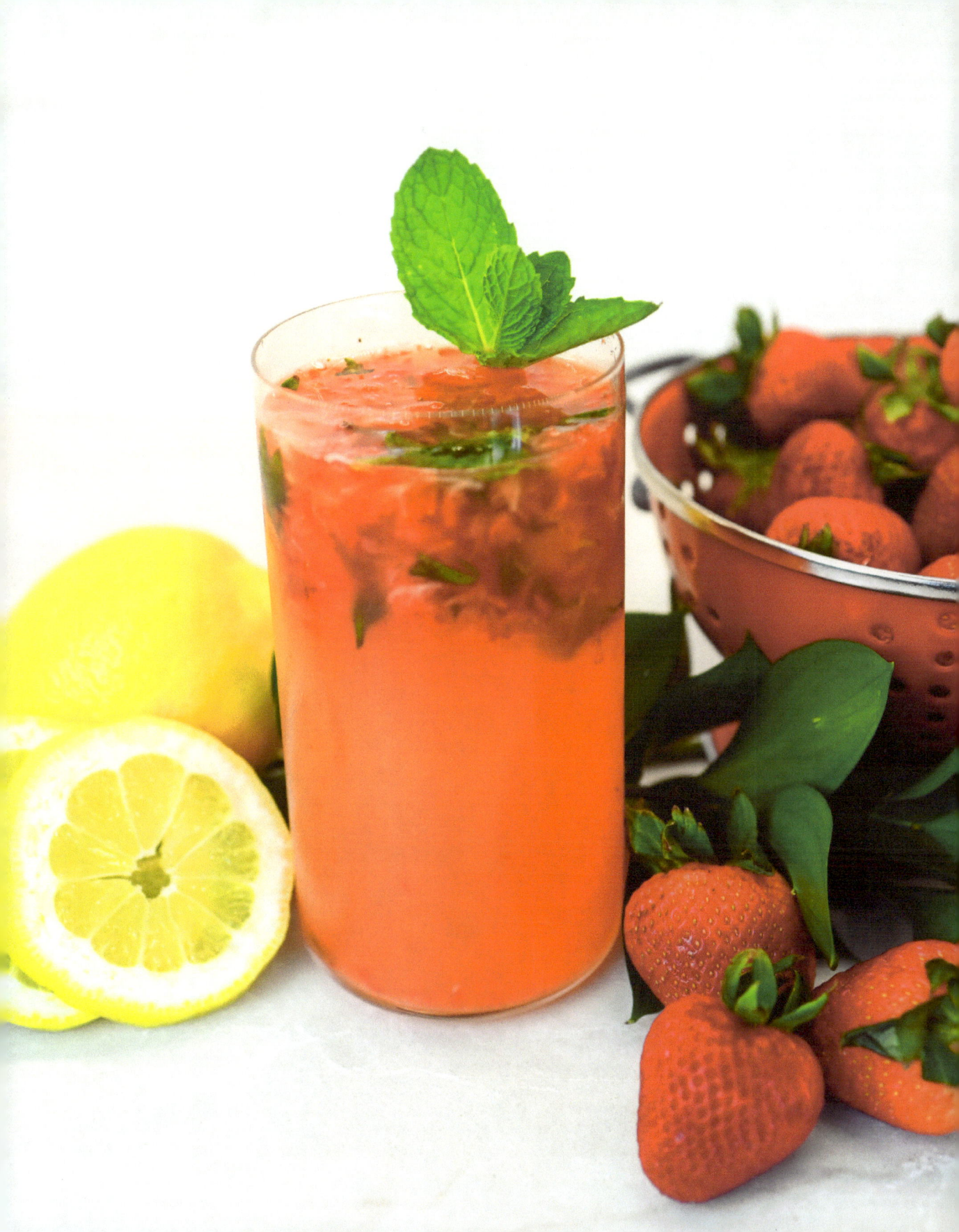

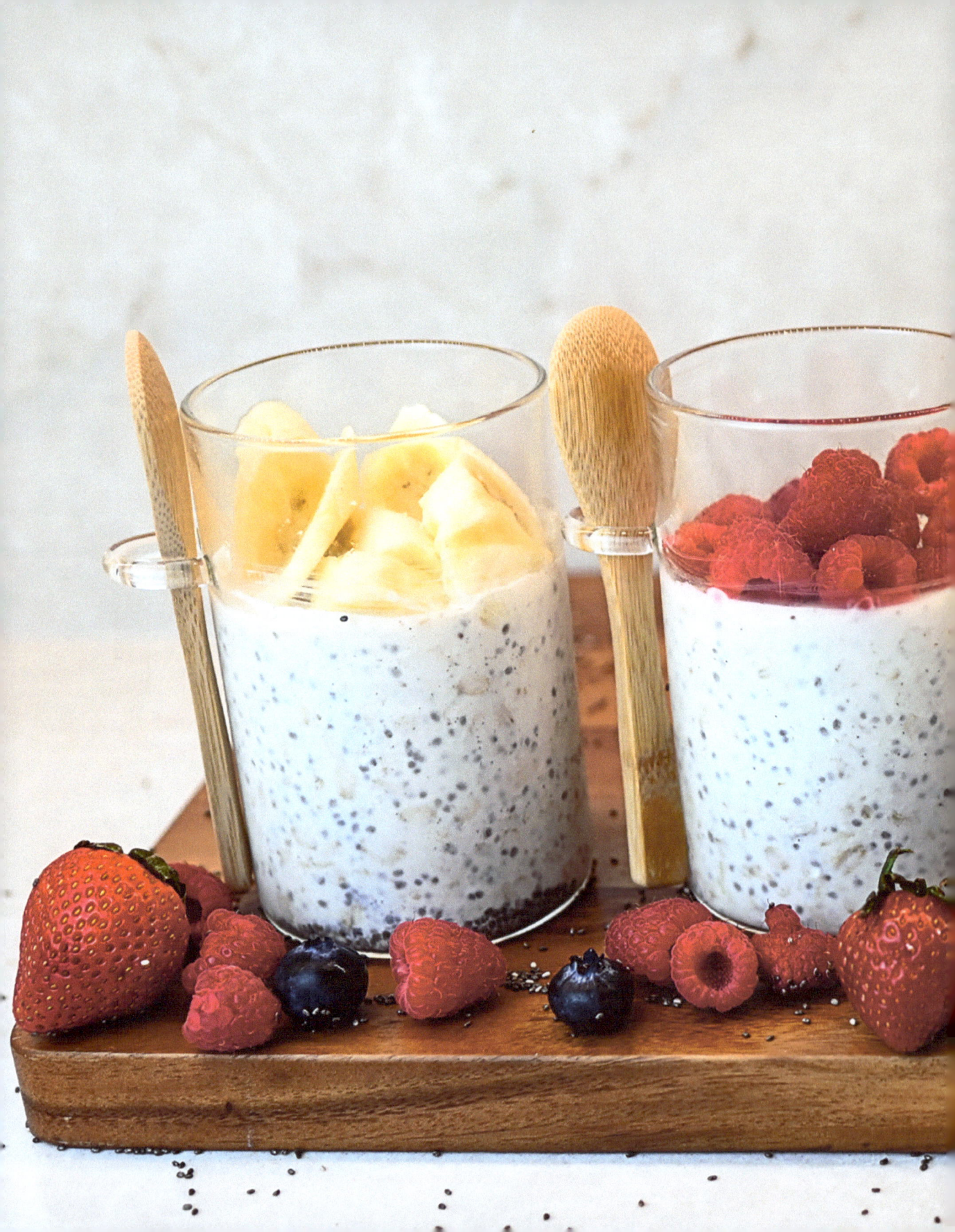

bites & delights

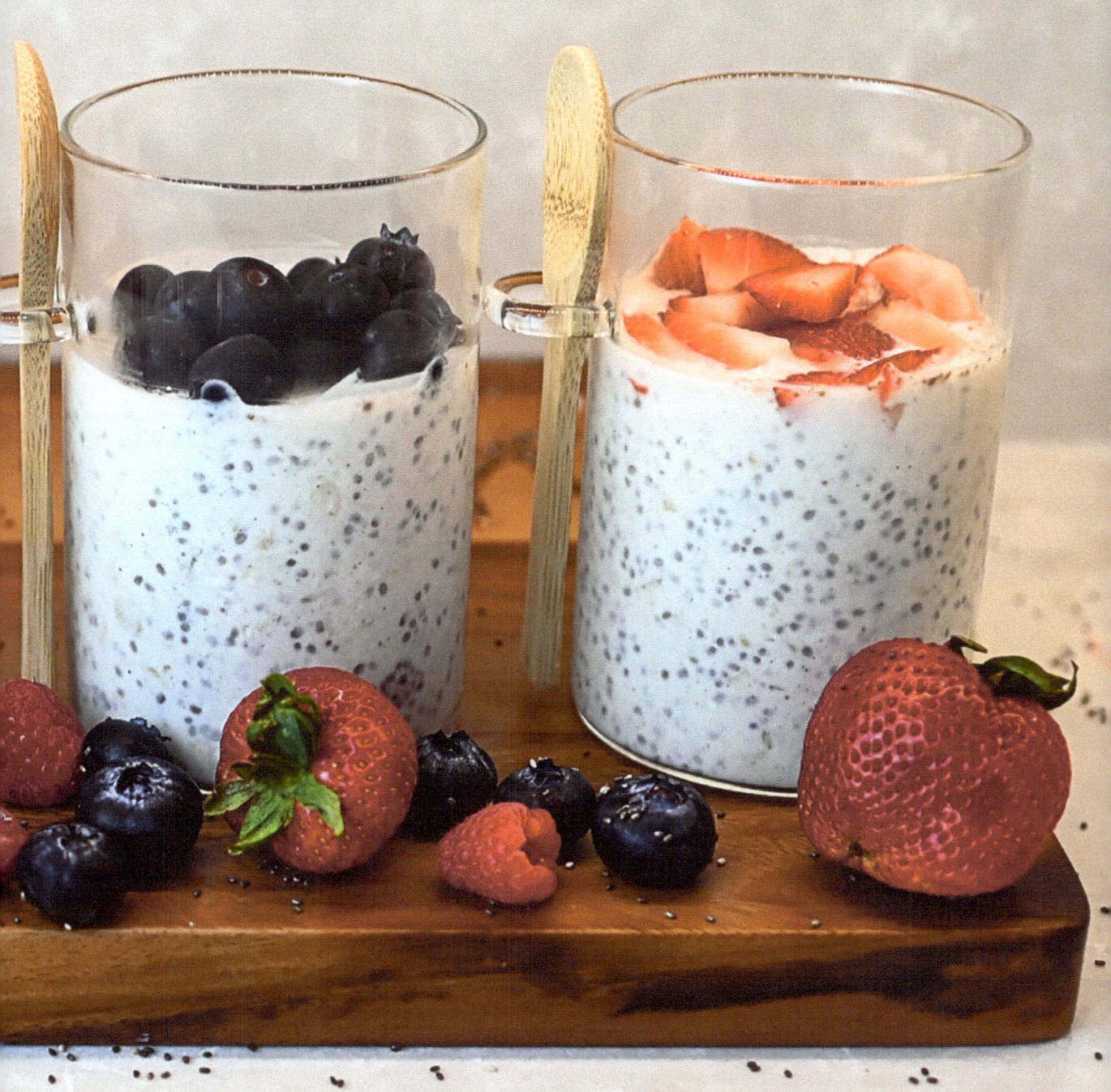

almondmilk

Ingredients

------ ------

- 1½ cup almonds
- 4 cups filtered water
- 4 pitted dates
- ¼ teaspoon cinnamon
- ½ teaspoon vanilla extract
- dash of salt

Instructions

------ ------

1. Soak almonds in water overnight at least 8 hours
2. Strain water
3. Put almonds in high-speed blender with 4 cups of filtered water
4. Add dates, cinnamon, vanilla, and salt
5. Blend in high-speed blender for 1 minute or until fully blended
6. Strain milk through cheesecloth bag, squeezing out at the end.
7. Add more cinnamon and/or vanilla to taste
8. Put in glass storage container and refrigerate immediately
9. Consume within 3 days for freshness

TIP

 Nut Milk Makers are all the rage these days. They make smaller ones for home use, and Holly finds them to be very efficient. They cut out the need for a cheesecloth bag and you can use a fine mesh strainer instead. It also cuts out the time of needing to soak the almonds in advance.

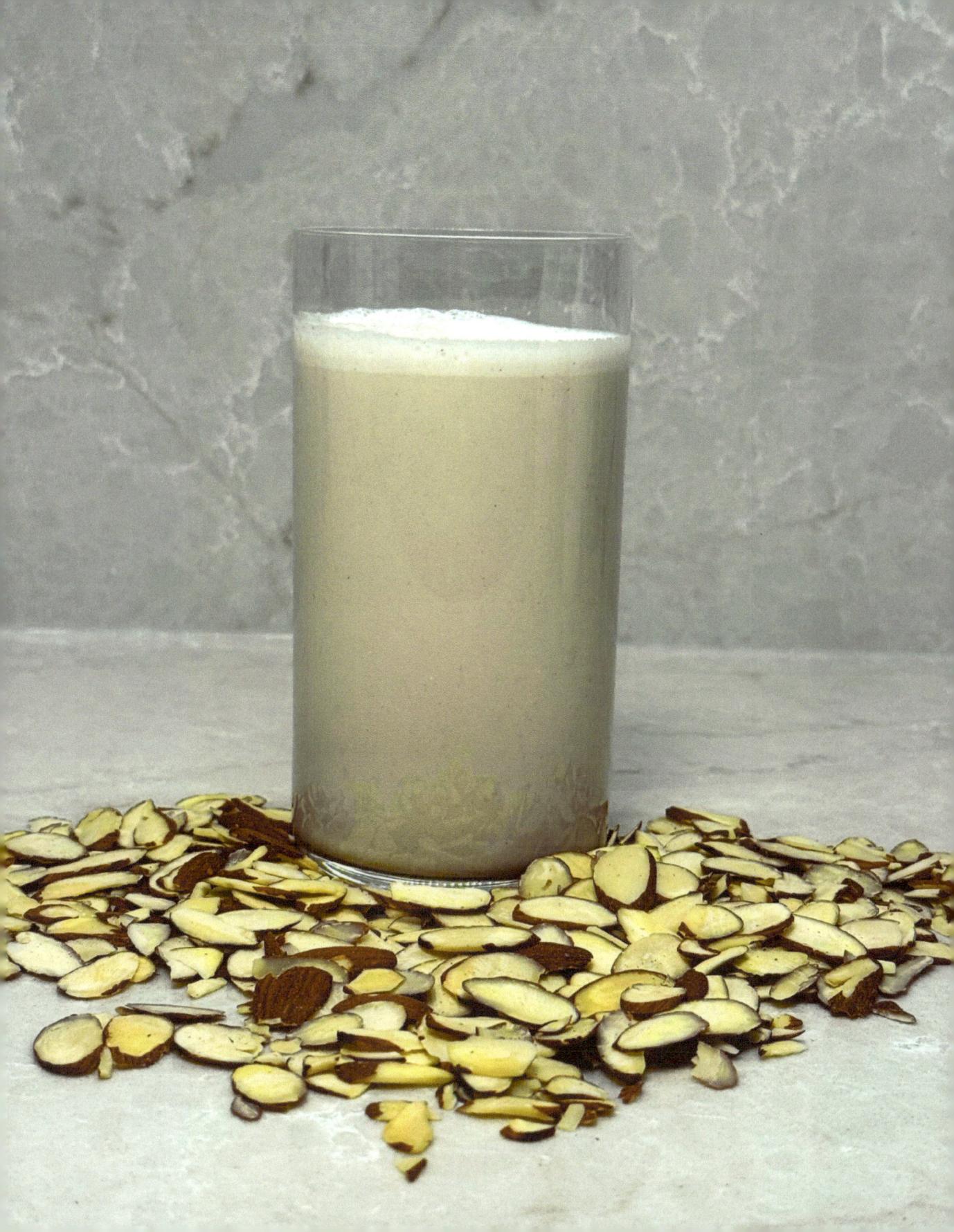

bananachiaseedpudding

yield: about 3 8-ounce containers

Ingredients

- 2 cups (16 ounces) unsweetened almond milk
- ¼ cup chia seeds
- 1 teaspoon of pure vanilla extract
- 1 teaspoon of Ceylon cinnamon powder
- 1 ripe banana

Instructions

1. Add all ingredients in a blender and mix until smooth.
2. Best chilled overnight. Chill for at least 1 hour.
3. Use topping of your choice.

Use homemade almond milk. Yum!

ADD INS/TOPPINGS

 Berries (strawberries, blueberries, raspberries, pineapple, kiwi), shredded coconut, Goji berries, or dark chocolate.

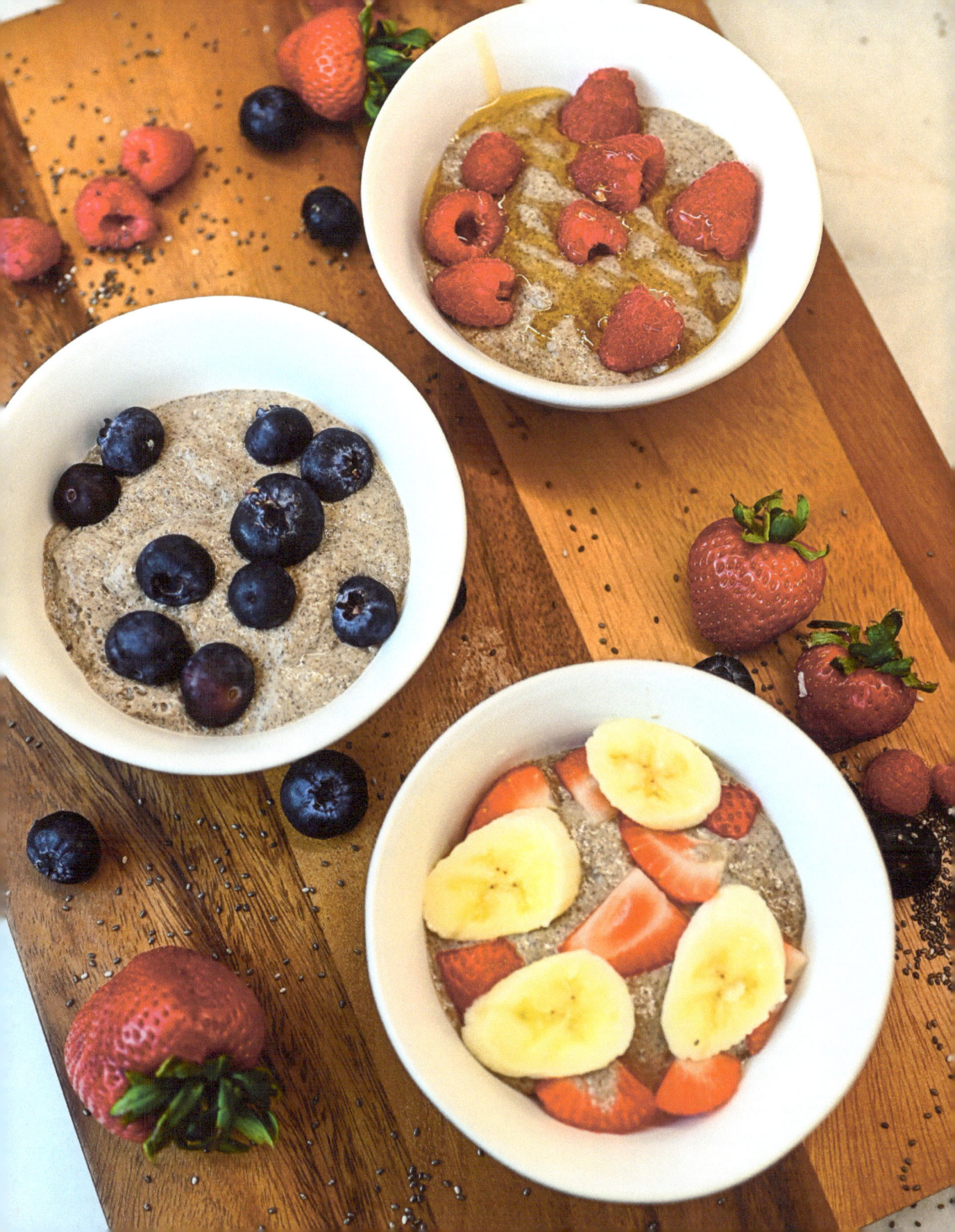

bananaoatenergybites

These no-bake energy bites are naturally sweet, satisfying, and perfect for a quick snack or breakfast on the go!

Ingredients

- 2 ripe bananas
- 2 cups rolled oats
- ¼ cup almond butter
- ¼ cup honey
- 2–3 tablespoons protein powder (optional)
- 1 tablespoons chia seeds
- 2 tablespoons mini dark chocolate chips
- ½ teaspoon Ceylon cinnamon

Instructions

1. In a large mixing bowl, mash the ripe bananas until smooth.
2. Add the rolled oats, almond butter, honey, chia seeds, protein powder, chocolate chips, and cinnamon to the bowl.
3. Stir everything together until fully combined.
4. Chill in the fridge for 20 minutes. If the mixture feels too wet, add a few more oats as needed.
5. Using clean hands or a small scoop, roll the mixture into small balls, about 1 inch in diameter.
6. Store in the refrigerator in an airtight container for a convenient, ready-to-eat snack any time!

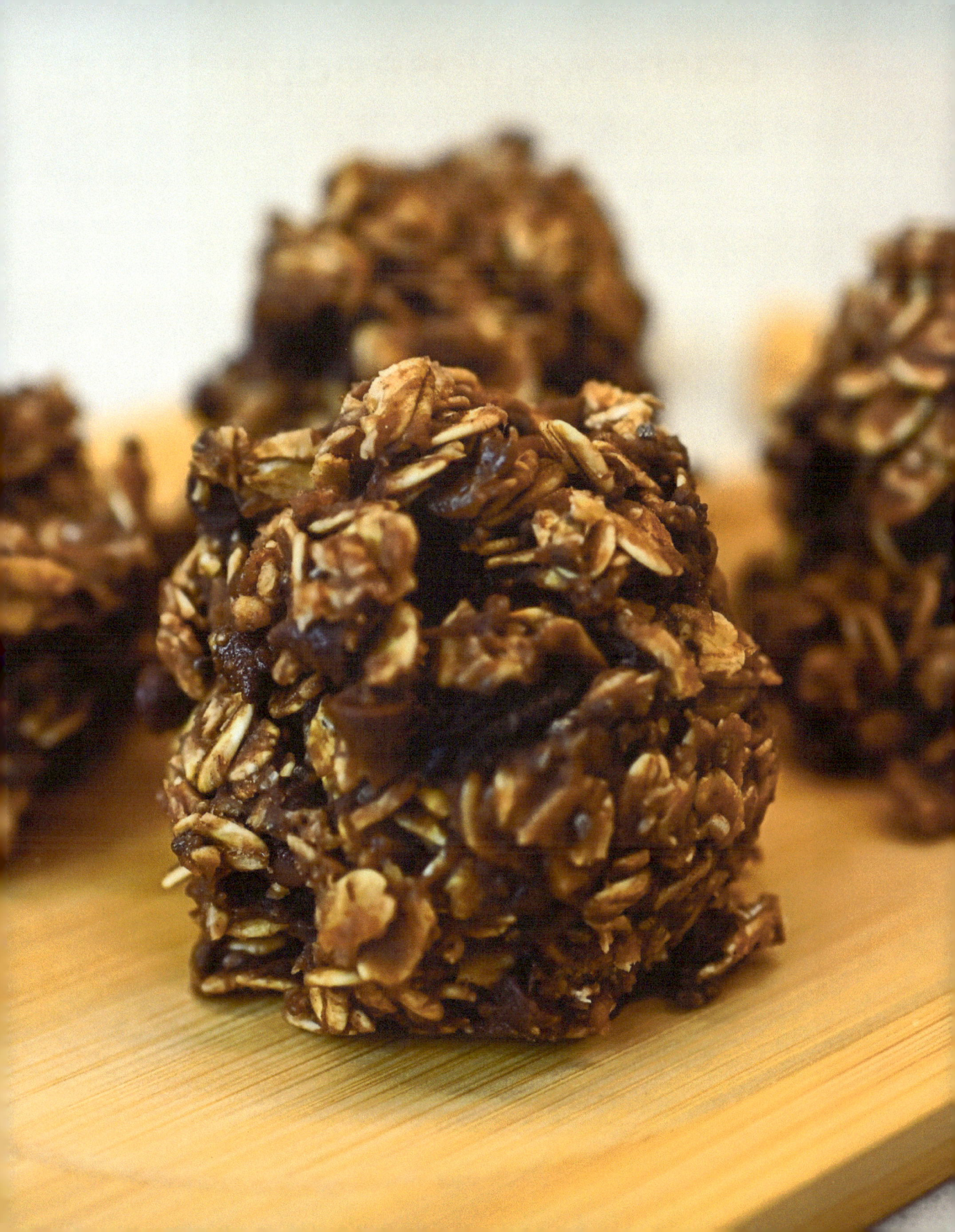

cashewchiaseedpudding

yield: about 5 8-ounce containers

Ingredients

- 2 cups (16 ounces) unsweetened almond milk
- 8 ounces water
- 1.5 cups of raw cashews
- ¼ cup chia seeds
- 4 dates
- 1 teaspoon of pure vanilla extract
- 1 teaspoon of Ceylon cinnamon

Instructions

1. Add all ingredients in a blender and mix until smooth.
2. Best chilled overnight. Chill for at least 1 hour.
3. Use topping of your choice.

Use homemade almond milk. Yum!

ADD INS/TOPPINGS

 Berries (strawberries, blueberries, raspberries, pineapple, kiwi), shredded coconut, Goji berries, or dark chocolate.

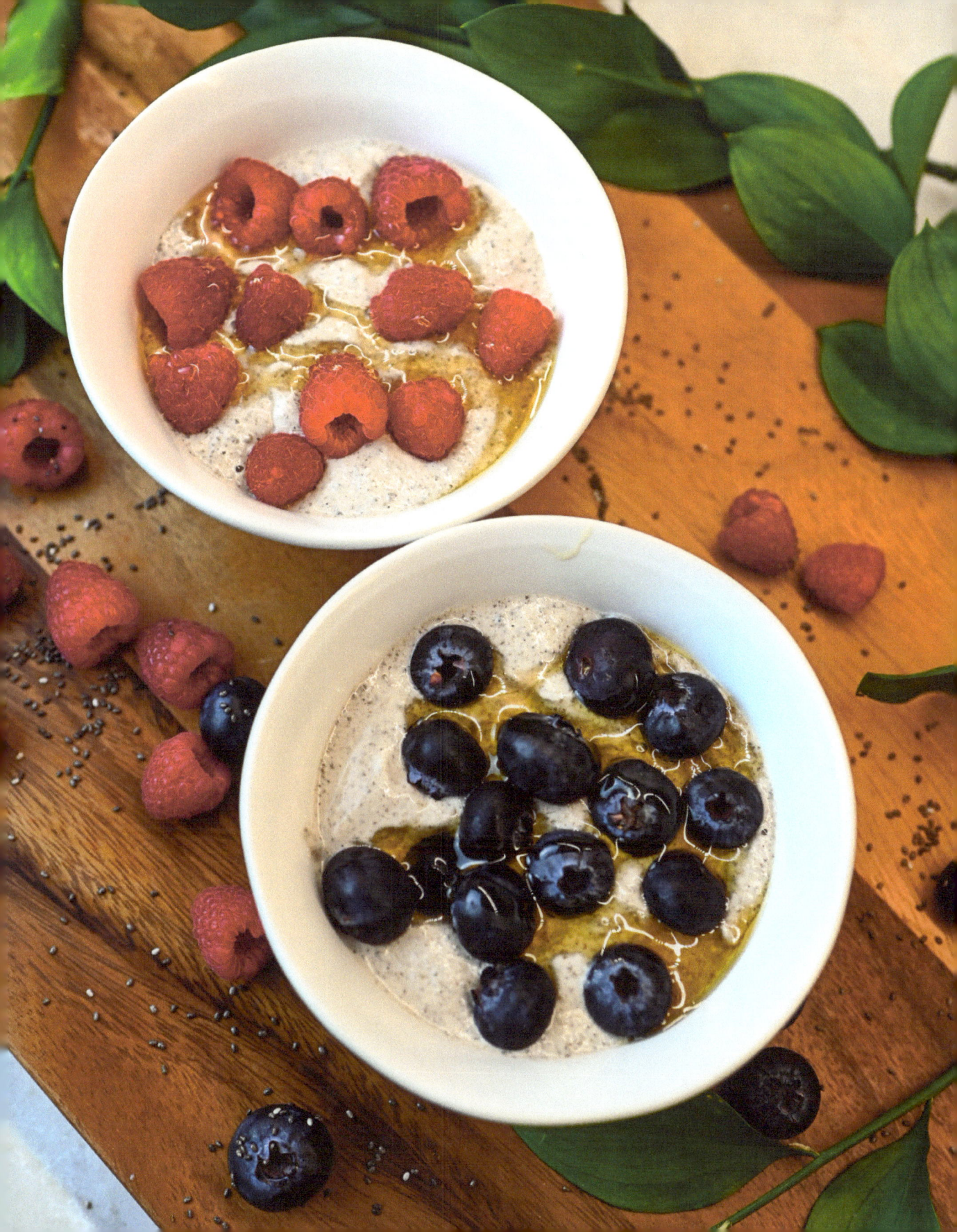

darkchocolate pistachiobites

Ingredients

Base:

- 20 dates (pitted)
- 1/2 cup dry roasted pistachios
- 1/2 cup raw pumpkin seeds
- 1/2 cup almond butter

Toppings:

- 1/4 cup chopped pistachios (set aside from above)
- 2 tablespoons raw pumpkin seeds
- Sprinkle of sea salt flakes
- 1.5 cups dark chocolate (for melting)

Instructions

1. Prep your pan: Line an 8x8" dish with parchment paper.
2. Melt the chocolate: In a double boiler or microwave (short intervals, stirring often), melt the dark chocolate until smooth. Set aside.
3. Chop pistachios for topping: In a food processor, pulse ¼ cup pistachios until roughly chopped. Set aside for topping.
4. Make the base mixture: In the food processor, combine: dates, remaining pistachios, pumpkin seeds, and almond butter. Blend until thick and sticky, scraping down the sides as needed.
5. Form the base layer: Press the mixture evenly into your prepared pan.
6. Add chocolate layer: Pour and spread the melted chocolate evenly over the base.
7. Add toppings: Sprinkle with chopped pistachios, pumpkin seeds, and a pinch of sea salt flakes.
8. Initial chill: Freeze for 15 minutes to set the chocolate.
9. Cut into pieces: Remove from freezer, slice into desired bite-size pieces, then return to the pan.
10. Final chill: Freeze again for 45 minutes until firm.
11. To serve: Let bites sit at room temperature for about 5 minutes before eating.
12. Storage: Store in an airtight container in the freezer.

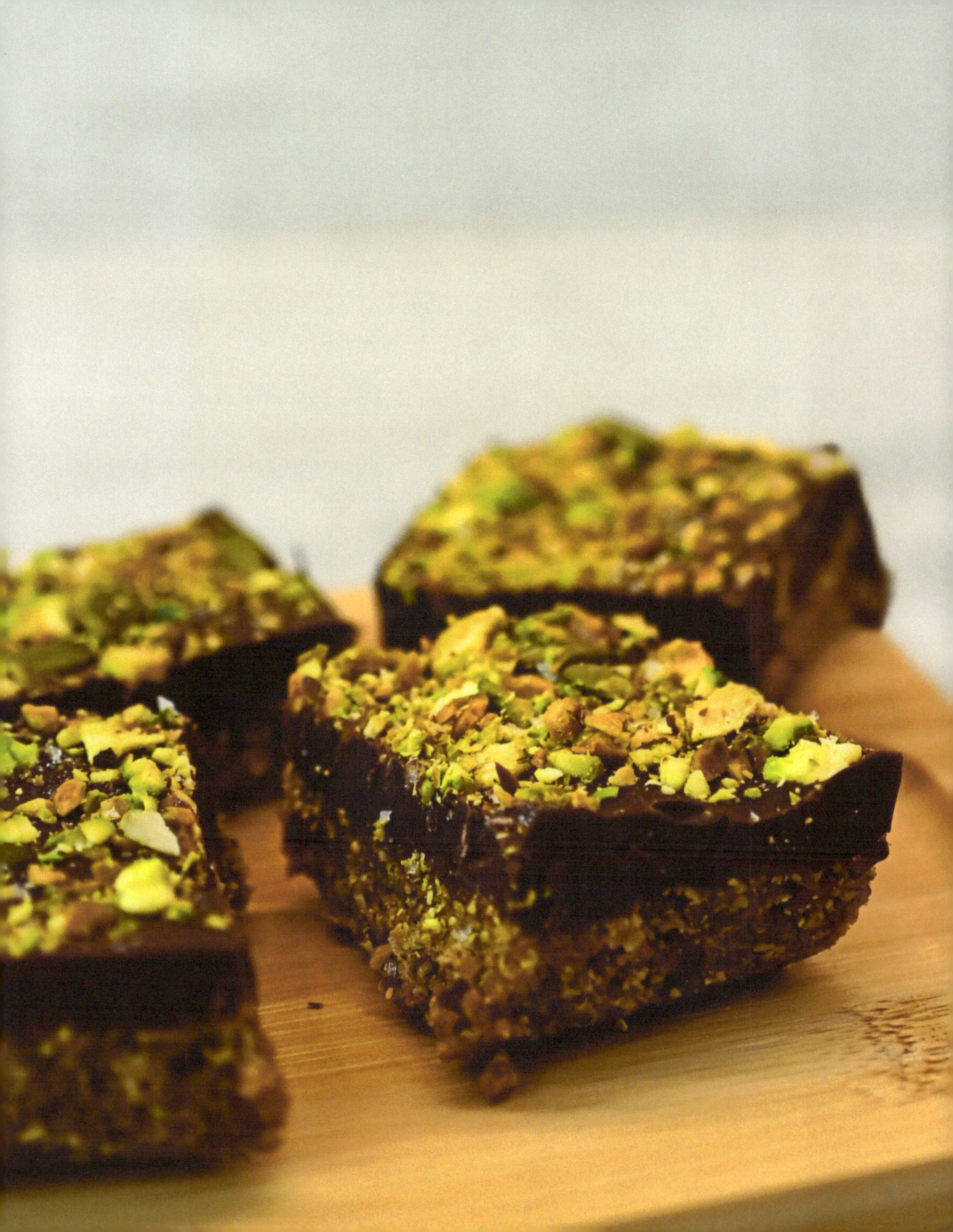

darkchocolate superfoodbites

A nutrient-packed, delicious treat made with dark chocolate, almond butter, and a mix of super seeds. Perfect for a quick energy boost or a healthy dessert!

Instructions

1. Prep your pan: Line an 8x8" dish with parchment paper.
2. Melt the chocolate: In a double boiler or microwave (short intervals, stirring often), melt the dark chocolate until smooth.
3. Pour and spread a thin layer of melted chocolate evenly across the bottom of the dish.
4. Evenly layer the halved dates over the chocolate.
5. Spoon and gently spread the almond butter over the dates.
6. In a small bowl: Mix together the chia seeds, pumpkin seeds, and hemp seeds.
7. Sprinkle half of the seed mixture evenly over the almond butter.
8. Pour and spread the remaining melted chocolate over the top.
9. Sprinkle the rest of the seed mixture evenly on top.
10. Finish with a light sprinkle of sea salt.
11. Place in the freezer for about 1 hour, or until completely set.
12. Once frozen: Remove from the dish and cut into bite-sized squares.
13. Store in the freezer for a convenient, grab-and-go treat.

Ingredients

- 1.5 cups dark chocolate, melted
- ½ cup almond butter
- 10 dates, halved
- 2 tablespoons chia seeds
- 2 teaspoon pumpkin seeds
- 2 tablespoons hemp seeds
- 1 teaspoon sea salt

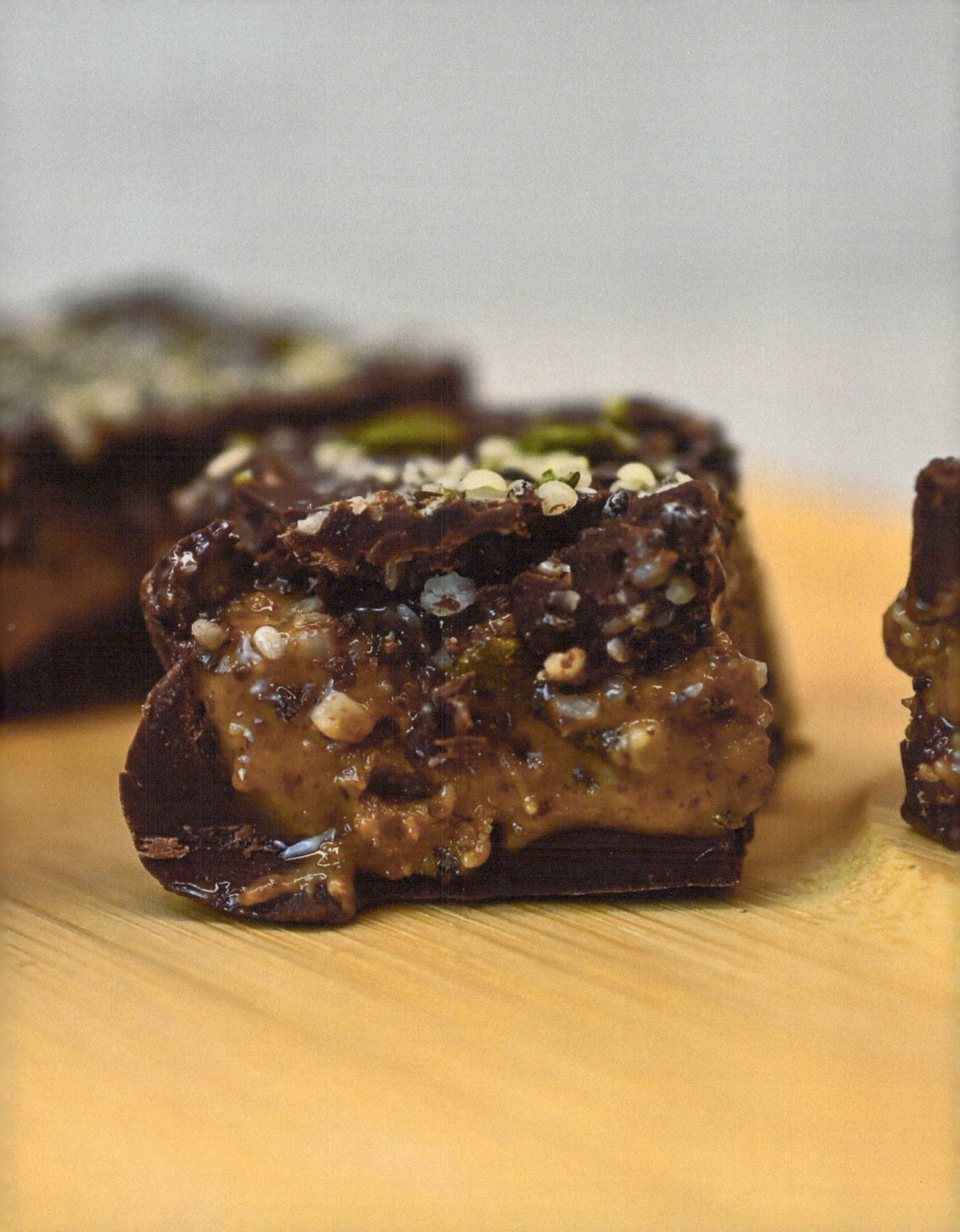

immuneboostpaste

Ingredients

small batch

- 2 tablespoons fresh ginger, finely grated or minced
- 1 tablespoon fresh turmeric, finely grated or minced
- 1 tablespoon fresh garlic, minced
- 1 teaspoon ground Ceylon cinnamon
- A pinch of black pepper (to help activate the turmeric)
- Honey to taste (start with 1–2 tablespoons)

large batch

- ½ cup fresh ginger
- ¼ cup fresh turmeric
- ¼ cup fresh garlic cloves, peeled
- 2 teaspoons ground Ceylon cinnamon
- ½ teaspoon black pepper
- ½ to ¾ cup raw honey (start with ½ cup)

A powerful, zesty blend of immune-supportive ingredients—perfect for stirring into warm water, tea, or adding to meals for a wellness boost. Or just eat it right off the spoon. **Use 1 teaspoon daily.**

Instructions

1. In a small bowl (or mini food processor if large batch), combine the ginger, turmeric, garlic, cinnamon, and black pepper.
2. Stir well (or pulse) to mix (chop) all the ingredients evenly.
3. Add honey gradually, mixing until it forms a thick, paste-like consistency. Adjust the amount of honey to suit your taste and desired texture.
4. Transfer to a clean, airtight jar and store in the refrigerator.

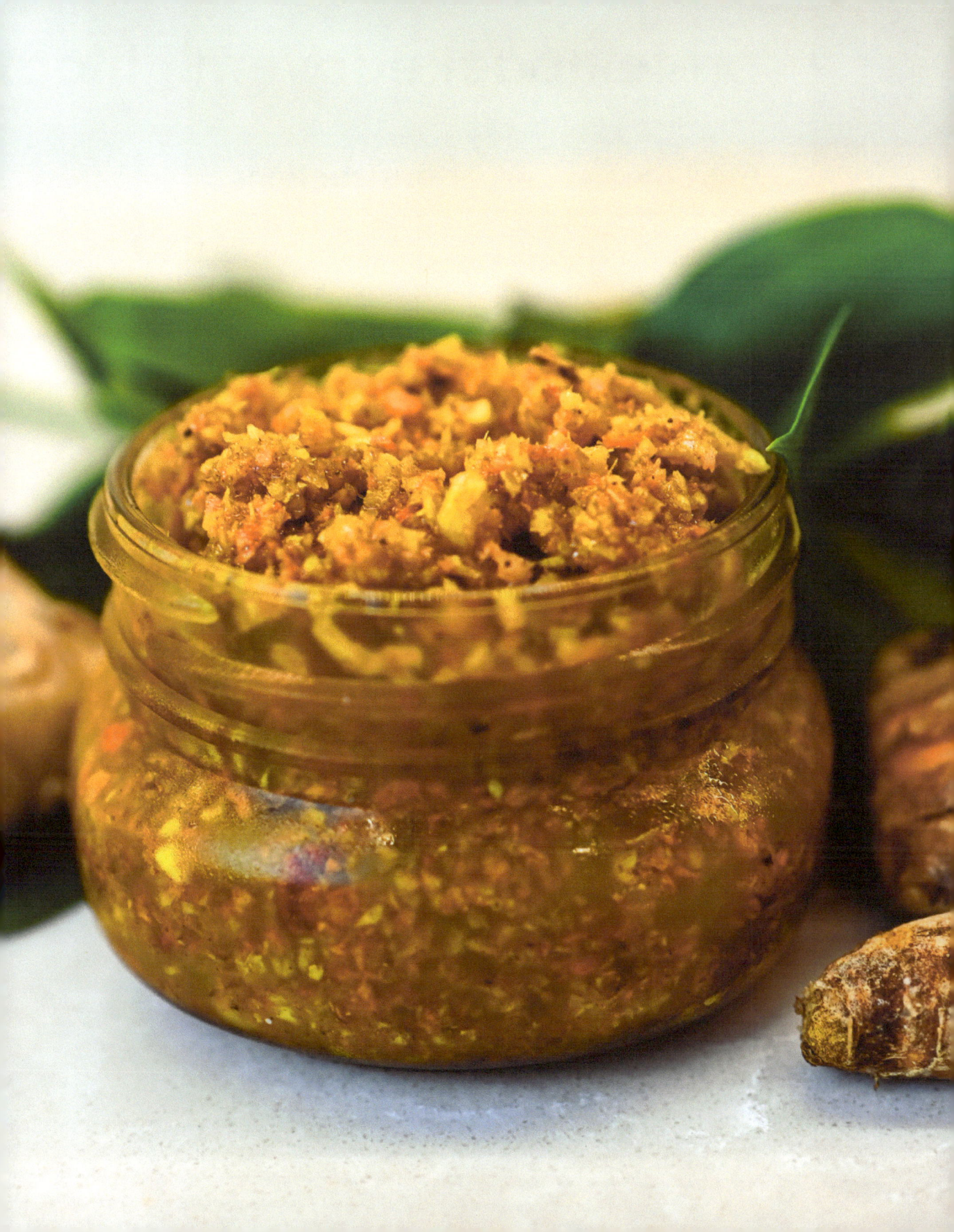

proteinpackedovernightoat

Ingredients

1 serving

- ½ cup rolled oats
- 1 tablespoon chia seeds
- ½ cup Greek yogurt (plain or flavored)
- 1 scoop protein powder (your choice of flavor)
- ¾ cup unsweetened almond milk

4 servings

- 2 cups rolled oats
- 4 tablespoons (or ¼ cup) chia seeds
- 2 cups Greek yogurt
- 4 scoops protein powder
- 3 cups unsweetened almond milk

Instructions

1. Mix the base: In a jar or container, combine oats, chia seeds, Greek yogurt, protein powder, and almond milk. Stir until well combined.
2. Add flavor (optional): Stir in any extras like cinnamon, vanilla, or a sweetener if desired.
3. Seal and chill: Cover and refrigerate overnight (or at least 4 hours) to let the oats and chia seeds absorb the liquid.
4. Top and enjoy: In the morning, give it a good stir and add your favorite toppings.

ADD INS/TOPPINGS

 Fresh fruit (bananas, berries, apples), nut butter (almond, peanut, cashew), honey or maple syrup (for sweetness), Ceylon cinnamon or pure vanilla extract, nuts, seeds, or granola (for crunch).

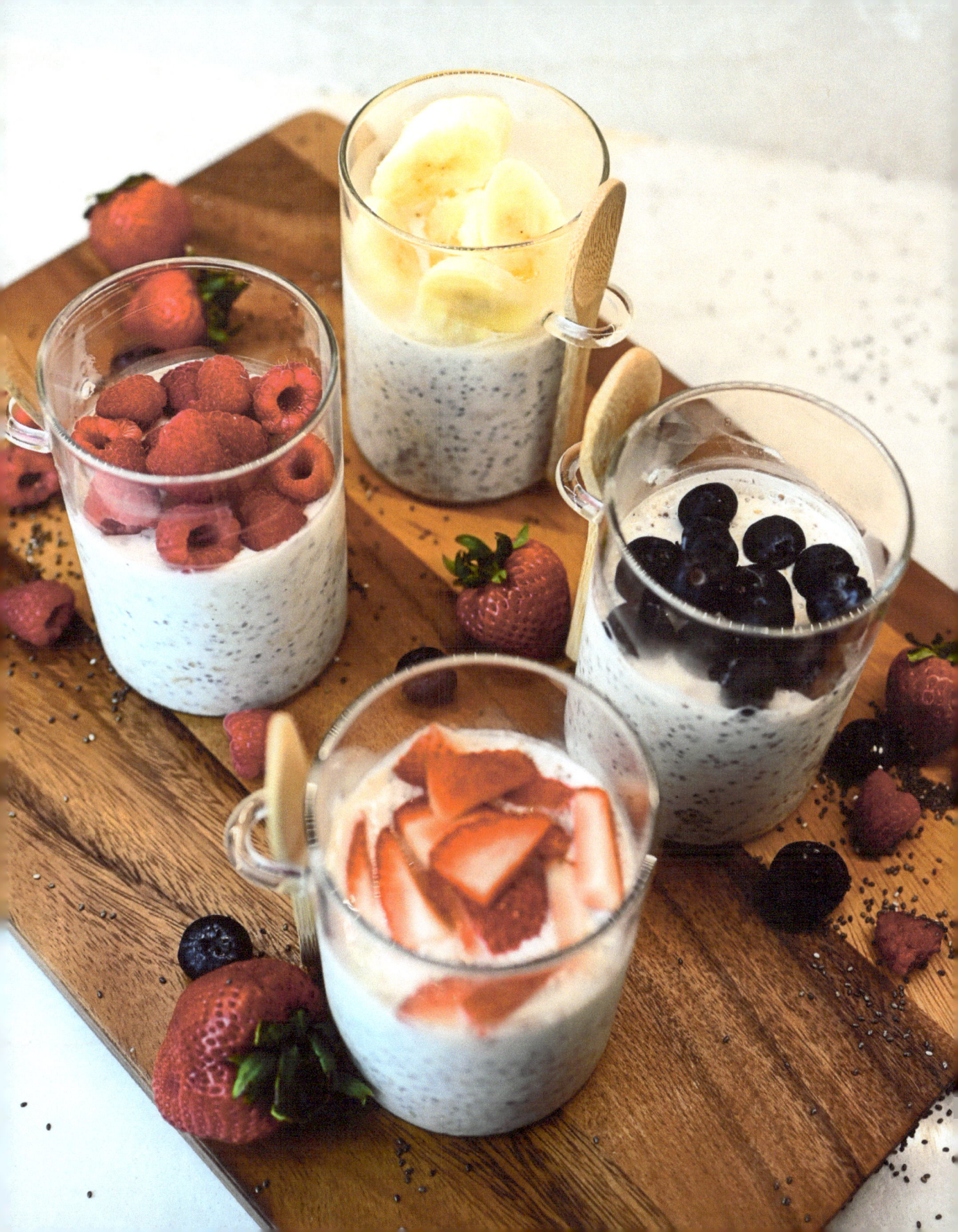

signatureicedcoffee

Ingredients

- 2 ounces maple syrup
- 5.5 ounces oat milk (just over ⅓ of the cup)
- 8.5 ounces iced coffee

Instructions

1. Prepare your preferred coffee and cool it.
2. Fill cup with ice.
3. Add maple syrup, iced coffee, & oat milk and stir.

TIP

 Drink with a straw so you can stir maple syrup around as you drink it.

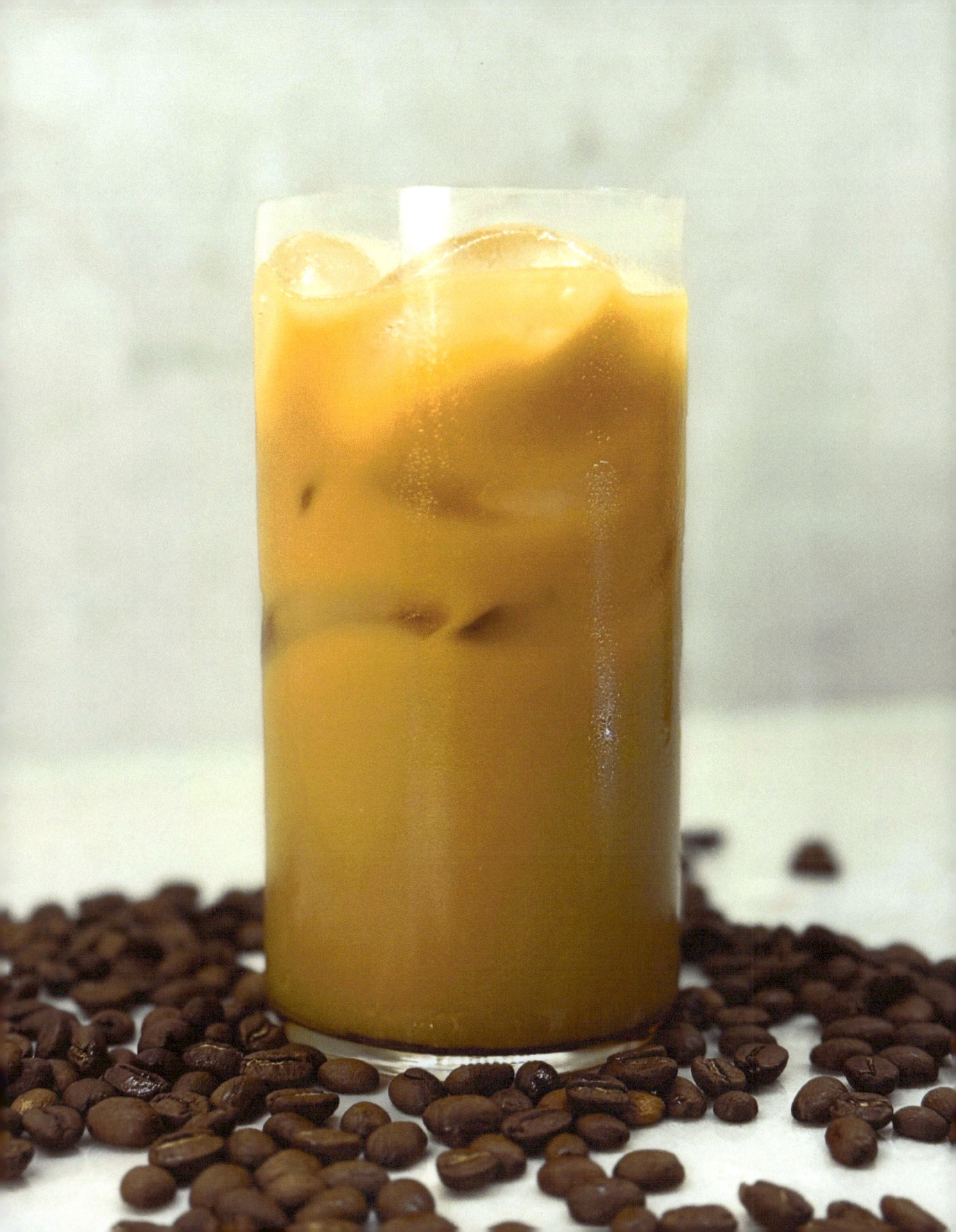

thebrazil

Ingredients

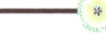

- 10 ounces iced coffee
- 6 ounces almond milk
- ½ cup raw cashews
- 2 dates
- ½ tablespoon of coconut flakes or cubes

Instructions

1. Add all ingredients into a blender and mix until smooth.
2. Store in the refrigerator.

This is Holly's all-time favorite drink with coffee.

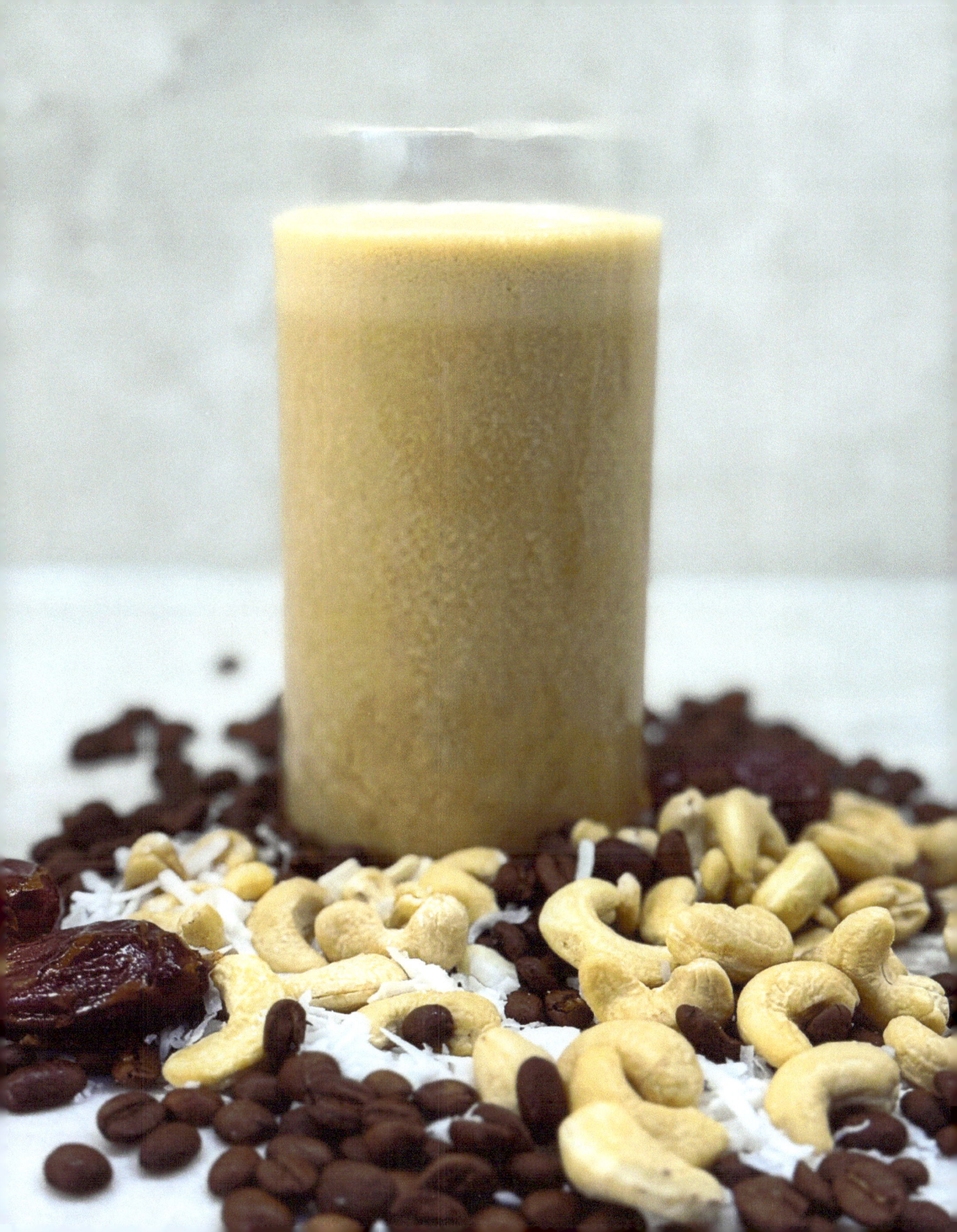

ACKNOWLEDGMENTS

To my son, Dylan — I'm so proud of you, your work ethic, and the incredible person you've become. I can't wait to see where life takes you.

To my husband, Robbie — I know you're relieved not to be on call anymore! Thank you for always knowing when to show up and save the day. Some of my favorite moments were listening to you handle the window—you always brought laughter. You're truly one of a kind.

To Christy — I only wish you had come to work at the café sooner. It's been an absolute pleasure. Thank you for your unwavering support and friendship.

To Celia — Thank you for being you. There's so much I could say, but I'll keep it short: It's definitely strawberry mint lemonade. You get it.

To Kas — I'm so lucky to have a friend like you. Thank you for being a constant and true presence in my life.

To Lauren — Some bonds are built in silence, and ours is one of them. Thankful for you.

To Chelsea from Represent Publishing — Thank you for taking on this project. You're truly great at what you do, and you have a magical way of calming my chaos. I've genuinely enjoyed our time working together . . . I guess I'll have to write another book just so we can hang out again!

ABOUT THE AUTHOR

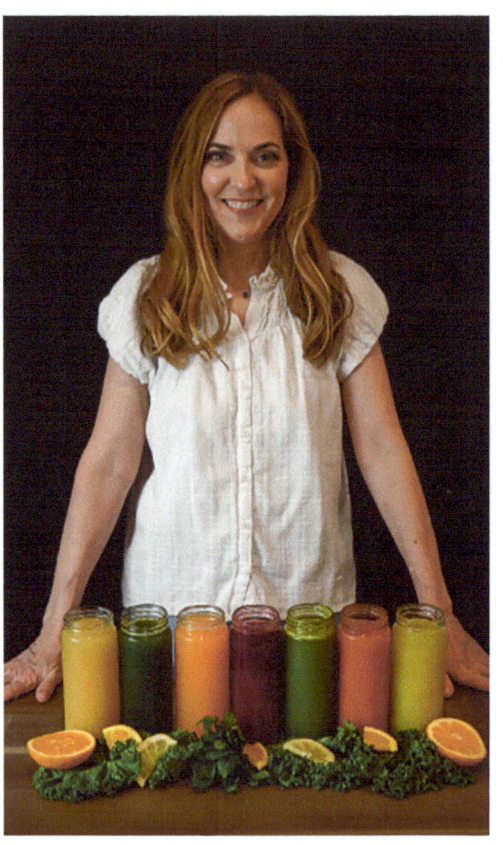

Holly's path to health and wellness is a true testament to the transformative power of personal growth and its ability to inspire others. Becoming a mother sparked Holly's commitment to creating a healthy home for her son, which led her to explore nutrition and well-being in depth. She found creative ways to incorporate more fruits and vegetables into his meals, along with establishing their daily smoothie routines. Holly's transition to vegetarianism and her pursuit of health coaching further solidified her dedication to this lifestyle. With over 20 years of business experience and a decade in the fitness industry—known for her energizing cycling classes and wholesome treats—Holly has motivated countless people.

When Holly took over Little Apple in 2019, she leveraged her experience and transformed it into Little Apple Café, which became a haven offering fresh juices, superfood smoothies, and açaí bowls for those seeking nourishment. Now, with her book, Holly invites you to bring a taste of Little Apple Cafe into your home, sharing her favorite recipes and spreading the joy of healthy living.